OCR Level 2 National

Certificate in

# Health and Social Care

**Liam Clarke**

**Mary Riley**

**Veronica Dougherty**

Published in 2004 by:
Nelson Thornes Ltd
Delta Place
27 Bath Road
CHELTENHAM
GL53 7TH
United Kingdom

05 06 07 08 / 10 9 8 7 6 5 4 3 2

A catalogue record for this book is available from the British Library

ISBN 0 7487 8512 4

Illustrations by Barking Dog Art, Jane Bottomley, Angela Lumley and Alex Machin

Page make-up by Acorn Bookwork
Printed and bound in Great Britain by Scotprint

**Acknowledgements**

The authors and publishers are grateful to the following for permission to reproduce photographs and other copyright material in this book:

Liam Bailey, Photofusion p.253; Paul Baldesare, Photofusion pp.57, 58 (right) and 271; Sam Bird pp.221 (left) and 264. Thanks to Clare and Ian; John Birdsall pp.7, 66, 78, 79, 141 and 278; Paul Chitty, Photofusion p.279; Emily Dickinson p.223. Thanks to Rachel and Steve; Julia Martin, Photofusion pp.320; Brian Mitchell, Photofusion p.315; Molly Mulvihill p.151. Thanks to Caroline and Neil; Osprey/RMA p.74; Photodisc 40 (NT) p.224; Photodisc 59 (NT) p.322; RDK Mobility p.95; Martin Sookias pp.44, 66 and 155; Steve and Grace p.58 (left); Sure Start p.238.

Every attempt has been made to contact copyright holders, and we apologise if any have been overlooked. Should copyright have been unwittingly infringed in this book, the owners should contact the publishers, who will make corrections at reprint.

Cover photograph: Photodisc 18 (NT)

# Contents

# Preparing to give quality care

**1**

## To complete this unit you will need to:

- Illustrate how to support service users to maintain their rights
- Describe how service users' rights can be infringed and the responsibilities of care workers
- Recognise the diversity of service users and how to foster equality
- Recognise how to maintain confidentiality
- Review how legislation and policies help to maintain quality care
- Conduct a survey to investigate how a care setting maintains quality care.

 **AO1**    Illustrate how to support service users to maintain their rights

Service users have certain rights when using services or trying to gain access to them.

Many of these rights now are enshrined in charters and codes of practice but some are laid down by legislation, such as human rights and rights to be able to have access to GPs and hospitals for treatment.

Service users have a right to expect that you will:

- Identify and question your own values and prejudices, and their implications for practice
- Respect and value uniqueness and diversity, and recognise and build on strengths of the service user

1

- Promote and foster people's rights to choice, privacy, confidentiality and protection
- Assist people to increase control of, and improve the quality of, their lives
- Identify, analyse and take action to counter discrimination, racism, disadvantage, inequality and injustice
- Practise in a manner that does not stigmatise or disadvantage individuals, groups or communities
- Consult the service-user on all matters concerning their care.

## What other policies and procedures help you to support and maintain service users' rights?

### Charters

Many charters promote the rights of service users. Charters are very helpful because they tell the service user what they can expect from the service, how to complain about their support and what should happen when they complain.

Charters should clearly set out the principles and values that they are based on. These are:

- Treating service users with courtesy, honesty and respecting their dignity
- Helping service users to achieve and keep their independence
- Involving service users in making decisions and giving them enough information so that they can make informed choices
- Working in partnership with service users who need the services
- Helping service users to give their own views through advocacy and other representative organisations
- Making sure that service users feel they can complain about the services they receive and that this will not **negatively** affect the services they are getting
- Treating service users fairly on the basis of need and not discriminating against them on the basis of age, sex, race, religion, disability or sexual orientation.

Charters also contain:

- Information about the local services that are available and how to get them
- The standards that people can expect when they get services, information and advice
- The rules that decide if people can get help
- Information about how to complain if things are going wrong

- Targets for improvement and when these will be achieved
- Information about how people can say what they think about the services they are getting and how they can suggest ways of improving them
- Information about the charges people will be asked to pay
- Local telephone help line numbers and contact names, including local advocacy groups.

The Long Term Care Charter is an excellent example of a policy that supports service users' rights.

This national Long Term Care Charter tells anyone who needs long-term care or support the standards for the services that are provided and what to do if these expectations are not met. These standards and other information are published in the local charters that local housing, health and social services draw up with the help of users, carers, voluntary organisations, advocacy groups and others. Local charters are published by social service departments and housing authorities.

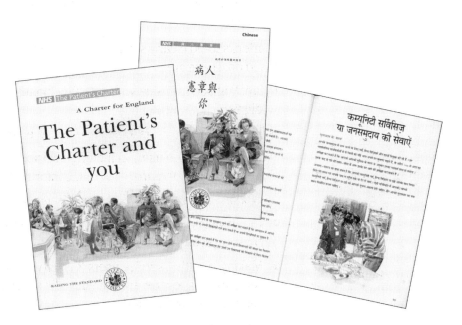

Local charters set out the standards and goals for improvement in six main areas. These are:

- Helping service users and carers to find out about services
- Understanding and responding to the needs of service users and carers
- Helping carers to care
- Finding a suitable place to live
- Helping people to stay independent
- Getting the right health care.

## Advocacy

Both care workers and service users, in order to contribute to the improvement of services, may require individual personal support and advice. For this reason, they will need to know where they may turn for guidance. In addition, some service users may require advocacy services. Advocacy is someone speaking for or acting on behalf of someone who may not be able to do so in person, in much the same way as a solicitor or barrister represents someone in court. While this is sometimes essential, who does the advocating remains an issue.

## Sources of support and guidance

There are numerous sources of support and guidance about issues relating to equality and rights available for care workers, service users and organisations. Much support is available on a national basis but help is sometimes even easier to obtain through local services. Support for equality of opportunity in general may be obtained from organisations such as the Commission for Racial Equality or the Equal Opportunities Commission. Local councils and trade unions also are significant sources of support and information.

As a consequence of the NHS and Community Care Act 1990, all local authorities have had to produce clear procedures for complaints. In addition, the annual community care plans that must be jointly produced with health authorities have to clearly describe the rights of service users. It is likely, however, that many service users remain unaware of these local public documents, so efforts should be made to make them more widely available.

Examples of some of the larger national sources of help and support relating to issues of equality and rights are described below.

### Equal Opportunities Commission

The Equal Opportunities Commission is the expert body on equality between women and men in the UK. It was created by Parliament in 1976 with three main tasks:

- Working to end sex discrimination
- Promoting equal opportunities for women and men
- Reviewing and suggesting improvements to the Sex Discrimination Act and the Equal Pay Act.

One of the most important functions of the Equal Opportunities Commission is to advise individuals of their rights and to encourage people to exercise them.

### Commission for Racial Equality

The Commission for Racial Equality is a publicly funded, independent organisation that exists to tackle racial discrimination and promote racial equality.

- It works in both the public and private sectors to encourage fair treatment and to promote equal opportunities for everyone, regardless of their race, colour, nationality, or national or ethnic origin.
- It provides information and advice to people who think they have suffered racial discrimination or harassment.
- It works with public bodies, businesses and organisations from all sectors to promote policies and practices that will help to ensure equal treatment for all.
- It runs campaigns to raise awareness of race issues and encourage organisations and individuals to play their part in creating a just society.
- It makes sure that all new laws take full account of the Race Relations Act and the protection it gives against discrimination.

### National Disability Council

The National Disability Council is an independent body with statutory duties to advise the Secretary of State for Education and Employment, when asked to do so or on its own initiative, in the following key areas:

- The elimination of discrimination against disabled people
- Measures to reduce or eliminate such discrimination
- The operation of the Disability Discrimination Act 1995.

The National Disability Council is charged with preparing:

- Proposals for a Code of Practice on the rights of access to goods, facilities, services and premises
- An annual report for Parliament at the end of each financial year.

### Disability Rights Commission

The UK government is committed to developing comprehensive and enforceable civil rights for disabled people. In October 1997 the government announced that it would:

- Set up a ministerial task force to report to the government on how best to secure those rights
- Implement the remaining provisions of the Disability Discrimination Act
- Establish a Disability Rights Commission.

### The Council of Europe

The Council of Europe is an international organisation based in the French city of Strasbourg. Its main role is to strengthen democracy, human rights and the rule of law throughout its member states. The defence and promotion of these fundamental values is no longer simply an internal matter for governments but has become a shared and collective responsibility of all the countries concerned.

### National Association of Citizens' Advice Bureaux

The aims of the Citizens' Advice Bureau are:

- To ensure that individuals do not suffer through lack of knowledge of their rights and responsibilities or of the service available, or through an inability to express their needs effectively and, equally,

- To exercise a responsible influence on the development of social policies and services, both locally and nationally.

The four principles of Citizens' Advice are:

- Independence
- Confidentiality
- Impartiality
- Free.

### MIND

MIND campaigns for the right to lead an active and valued life in the community and is an influential voice on mental health issues. Local MIND associations offer many services, including supported housing, crisis helplines, drop-in centres, counselling, befriending, advocacy, employment and training schemes around the country.

MindinfoLine offers thousands of callers every year vital confidential help on a range of mental health problems and their consequences.

MIND advises the government, health and local authorities and the public on good practice, services and developments in mental health and community care. MIND's policies are always developed in consultation with the MindLink user network and allied organisations.

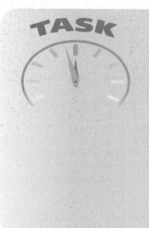

## TASK

### How to support service users and maintain their rights

To complete the assignment you should gather information from as many sources as possible. It would be helpful if you interviewed carers and service users and read as widely as possible.

You should identify and write about three rights that service users have, such as the right to have their own GP, to confidentiality, to protection, to equal and fair treatment and to be consulted on matters affecting themselves.

Give three detailed examples of how care workers could apply the three rights that you have identified in a care setting.

### Trade unions

Another very important source of support is the trade union. Many trade unions fight for the rights of their members and oppressed groups in general. Workers in health and social care services make much use of their unions (UNISON being the major source of advice and support).

AO2 ## Describe how service users' rights can be infringed and the responsibilities of care workers

Essentially, service users should have the same choices and rights as are afforded to all of us in everyday life. This means that service users' wishes and preferred responses to them should be encouraged, listened to, acknowledged and recorded.

## Individual rights and choice – personal

Options, rather than solutions, should be presented to the service user, and the differences among the options should be fully explained. Options should always be considered in respect of risk but only in exceptional circumstances should the right to take risks be removed from the service user. Most commonly, such a situation may arise when it is felt that the service user cannot make a reasonable assessment of the risk, for instance in a case of mental illness or severe learning disability. In such a case, the service user's rights are legally protected by the Mental Health Act 1983.

*In the busy working day, it is easy to forget a service user's individual identity and rights*

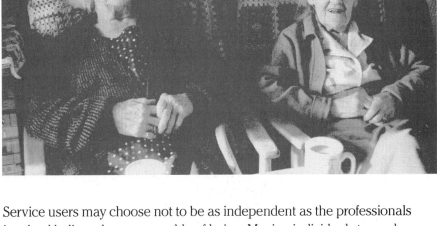

Service users may choose not to be as independent as the professionals involved believe they are capable of being. Moving individuals towards independence can only be done by encouragement: the right of individuals

to choose their preferred level of independence is what is important. For example, older people may wish more to be done for them because they choose not to push themselves. This process of disengagement is not unusual.

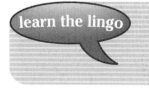

**Disengagement** means withdrawing and becoming less involved.

Carers must not only develop tolerance towards different types of individual but must also actively promote and support individual rights and choice. This requires good interpersonal skills.

Although it is possible to express values in care in fairly clear terms, putting values into practice is highly problematic. Real-life situations rarely present themselves in such clear-cut ways. Who should determine the best interests of service users?

### Individual rights and choice – physical

Service users' physical rights may be infringed if carers attempt to restrain them. This may happen if service users are confused, show challenging behaviours or need treatment under the Mental Health Act. It is important that carers do not attempt to use restraint without appropriate training.

No service user should have their physical rights infringed except in situations when it is specifically permitted by law, such as when they need psychiatric treatment or are a danger to themselves or other people.

### Individual rights and choice – financial

How can a service users financial right be infringed?

It is the responsibility of all carers to enable service users to administer their own financial affairs. This kind of action empowers service users and encourages them to take as much responsibility as possible for managing their own lives.

You should never assume that a service user needs assistance – always discuss the situation with them and allow them to make or contribute to any decisions that are necessary.

You may also infringe a service user's financial rights by not informing them of support services and allowances that are available to help them with their financial affairs, such as disability living allowance, invalid care allowance and incapacity benefit.

When working with families and other interested parties, it may be unclear how to balance the needs of all in an attempt to define the best interests of the service user.

*Seeking advice from colleagues*

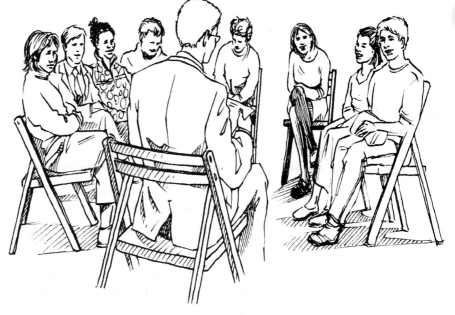

### The responsibilities of care workers – seek advice and guidance

It is the responsibility of all professional carers, when in doubt about the best interests of the service user, to seek advice from their line manager. Care workers also have a responsibility to work within the agency's policies and procedures and any guidelines or regulations laid down by their professional organisation.

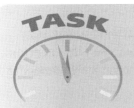

**TASK**

## How service users' rights could be infringed in care settings

Write three short, detailed scenarios showing how service users'

- Personal rights
- Physical rights
- Financial rights

can be infringed. It is important that you consider in particular how poor practice can lead to infringement of rights.

You should also identify three examples of good practice, as applied in care settings, that show how care workers apply their responsibilities in seeking advice and guidance from line managers and supervisors. You should also show policies that care workers use and procedures of professional organisations.

**AO3** # Recognise the diversity of service users and how to foster equality

## Personal values and attitudes

Much of our interpersonal interaction is guided by our personal values and attitudes. What we think is right and true affects the way we behave. Many of the ideas and assumptions we have are based on what we were told as children and later on what we have seen and heard on television or read about. Sometimes our own prejudices or personal fears and values are more subtle but are still significant in affecting how we relate to people.

All health and care workers must ensure that their attitudes and values do not influence their behaviour, which would undermine attempts to foster equality.

## Recognise diversity of service users

### Care values

Care values are principles, standards or qualities considered worthwhile or desirable by the care profession. These help us to recognise the diversity of service users and how to foster equality.

Three care values are:

- **Anti-discriminatory practice** – Not judging people because of their culture, race, religion, sexual identity, age, gender, health status, etc.
- **Confidentiality** – Service users have the right to say who should have access to personal data – care workers are responsible for respecting the wishes of the service user
- **Individual rights and choice, personal beliefs and identity** – Each individual's own personal beliefs and preferences – religious, cultural, political, ethical and sexual – must be respected.

The purpose of having care values is to create and foster equality and diversity for all individuals. While we emphasise the therapeutic, supportive and counselling roles of care workers, they are also responsible to the agency that they work for. A care worker may possess more power, through position, than their service user.

To foster diversity care workers have to know how to avoid discriminating against the culture, race, religion, sexual identity, age, gender or health status of the service user.

In their working practices, care workers must also take into account individual rights and choice. Service users' choice, preferences and wishes must be respected.

Service users' personal beliefs and identity must also be respected. This includes their religious, cultural, political, ethical and sexual beliefs.

To help you to maintain these values, listen to other individuals, promote effective communication in a variety of ways, consider service users' language (verbal and non-verbal) and understand their environment and social and cultural influences.

The social or health problems of some service users may create real dependency. To be seen as anything other than fit, able and making a valuable contribution to society is to be stripped of power. This is why we need to foster equality and individual rights and try to empower service users.

*Elderly people are largely written off as being of little use and dependent*

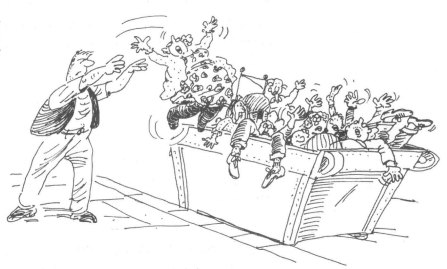

## Foster individual rights

Unless you treat each person as an individual you are likely to make assumptions about them – that is, to make a judgement about them based on something you have seen or read. The judgement may be wrong but it affects your interaction with that person. The assumption grows into a stereotype – we make the person fit the image we have of them rather than accepting them for what they are. Such stereotypes act as barriers to fostering service users' rights.

Good carers try to be aware of the stereotypes they may create, particularly when the person they are trying to help is from a different social class, a different ethnic background or the opposite gender. Here are some examples of how we can easily misjudge people and get the wrong message.

- **Gender –** We are socialised into our gender roles from the minute we are born, by the colour of the blanket that is wrapped around us and the sort of cards that are sent to greet us.
- **Age –** Negative stereotyping about age highlights sickness, dependency and not being able to be sociable. Older people or people with a disability may be seen by others as retarded, slow or inefficient.

- **Disability –** Often assumptions are made about disabled people's abilities based on misunderstanding. Access and opportunities are very significant to disabled people. If they are denied access to a building or the opportunity to do a job then they cannot demonstrate the capabilities they have. Similarly, socially some disabled people have experienced difficulties getting access to night clubs and other venues on the dubious grounds of increased fire risk.

## The basis of discrimination

The possible effects of discrimination are pervasive and wide-ranging. Reading novels, poems, watching films or television programmes and listening to personal experiences can inform you about the possible effects of discrimination.

Everyone stereotypes to a certain extent. We make judgements about people in our minds so that we can interact with them.

For example, if you met a young male wearing sports clothes you might assume he enjoyed playing sport. If you met a teenage girl wearing trendy clothes you might assume she liked listening to music and socialising. You might be very wrong in both cases but the misjudgements are probably not damaging.

When is stereotyping damaging and when does stereotyping become discrimination? These are not easy questions to answer because there may be only a subtle difference between stereotyping being helpful or being damaging to the other person. If you divide people into different categories you cannot assume that people who look or behave in a way that matches an image you have in your mind will fit into a particular category.

*What are your assumptions?*

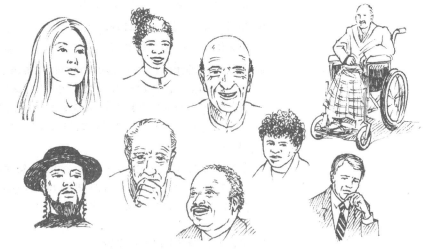

When people make assumptions like this we call it prejudice. It means someone has made up their mind beforehand what the person is going to be like. They have a personal bias, based on something they have heard or seen. It is confirmed and perpetuated in their response to people and their interactions with them.

Look at these comments – you can understand that there is prejudice and unhelpful categorisation in them:

- Only men should fly planes
- Only women make good nursery nurses
- People with disabilities shouldn't have children
- Lesbians and gays shouldn't teach in schools.

Sometimes articles or programmes can take a particular slant that categorises people in a certain way – as 'the Disabled' or 'the Old'. The article may be patronising (making the people seem like children) or give a lot of coverage to something a disabled person has achieved, however minor.

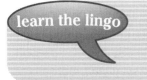

**learn the lingo**

While **prejudice** is what a person thinks, **discrimination** is what a person does – how they treat another person or group unfairly, based on their prejudice.

### Language

On a cultural level, our language is peppered with both sexist and racist terms that are indirectly discriminative. Often the words 'man', 'he' and 'him' are used to refer to both genders, for example 'chairman'.

## When can discrimination arise?

Prejudice or discrimination can arise at:

- An individual level, when people have personal attitudes and beliefs that they use to prejudge other groups negatively
- An institutional level, when the systems and practices of an organisation exclude certain groups from access to resources – for example, if publicity about antenatal classes was not produced in community languages in a multiracial area, this could be seen as institutional racism
- A cultural level, when people have so absorbed values, beliefs and ideas that they don't challenge negative stereotypes in media images. These people accept racist or sexist remarks.

## Types of discrimination

### Direct discrimination

There are obviously direct behaviours that are blatantly prejudiced, such as using offensive language, denying people rights or being rude. A young black girl was sitting on the inside seat of a bus. Her white friend, who was sitting beside her, stood up to let an older woman sit down. The woman refused the seat, saying she would rather stand than sit next to 'one of them'. The young black girl was the victim of direct discrimination.

### Indirect discrimination

Indirect discrimination is more subtle and less easy to report, but equally damaging. The senior manager who may have decided he doesn't want to appoint a female assistant manager may find ways of undermining her confidence (giving her menial jobs to do or always commenting that she is not competent) so that she doesn't even feel she can apply for the post. She becomes the victim of indirect discrimination.

Devaluing someone by not taking them seriously or not respecting what they say is a form of indirect discrimination. For example, assuming that everyone has a Christian name is a form of indirect discrimination.

### Racial discrimination

It is easy for black people or minority groups to be nudged out of healthcare services and therefore discriminated against almost by chance without people noticing. This may be because they are still relatively few in number. Similarly in schools, attitudes are set and may create tensions before any learning takes place. In the community, people are worried about employment and house sales and these fears are often directed against minority groups. Securing housing and employment therefore becomes more problematic for black people and, coupled with potential educational difficulties, such groups become disadvantaged through discrimination.

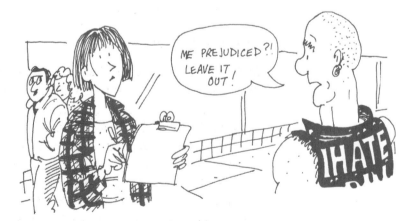

### Sexual discrimination

Research has shown that more people actually want sons than want daughters. Why do you think this might be?

People evidently have images of boy or girl children in their minds and what those male or female roles mean in life.

Think about the moment a child is born – Is it all right? Is it a boy or girl? The pink or the blue blanket covers the little body. The cards arrive conveying good wishes for the bouncing boy or the darling daughter. Soon, room decoration, clothes, toys, language, attitudes and responses all work to reinforce male or female roles. Later books, films, television programmes and expectations of relatives, parents and teachers may further confirm these roles. There doesn't seem anything wrong with this.

### Discrimination and disability

A similar process occurs in relation to mobility. It is easy to see a wheelchair or a white stick and categorise the person associated with them as being unable to cope. We may not even know what that person is capable of until further explanation.

## Effects of discrimination

Any kind of discrimination can cause damaging effects for those discriminated against. Discrimination can cause:

- Anxiety
- Depression
- Low self-esteem
- Loss of confidence
- Stress.

People who are discriminated against may also live in fear of others and may even suffer mental illness.

### People with a disability

Many disabled people feel that one of the worst aspects of being disabled is how other people see them. Very often it is assumed that disabled people cannot do things. For example, if someone is in a wheelchair there is a tendency for a speaker to address the person pushing the wheelchair rather than the person in the wheelchair. Of course, it is naive to suggest that a disabled person can do everything despite their disability, but if appropriate access, services and support are provided new opportunities can be opened up. There is also a lot of evidence of disabled people achieving physical and academic feats that some able-bodied people would never dream of.

Since 1970 all public buildings have by law had to provide wheelchair access. Similarly, pathways, walkways and staircases should not restrict wheelchair users. In reality, there are still enormous difficulties in terms of access. This limits disabled people socially and in the jobs they can get.

Similarly with housing: if a disabled person has an adapted home that they can manage this increases their independence. If funds are low and they have to rely on other people then they are limited.

### Effects of discrimination on children

If you are working with young children you can try to counteract stereotypical practices and language by:

- Encouraging role reversal – the boys play in the Wendy house and the girls with Lego (Is calling a playhouse 'the Wendy house' sexist?)
- Selecting books and posters reflecting positive images of black children and non-sexist attitudes
- Presenting toys and equipment in a non-sexist way
- Avoiding sexist, racist language yourself but also monitoring children's conversations
- Never saying things like 'Big boys don't cry' – it's probably better for the child to have a good bawl, male or female!
- Being firm about racist actions or language from children – act quickly to report it to a member of staff if you don't feel that it is appropriate for you to deal with it
- Not separating children on the basis of gender – grouping often sets up tensions and there is enough tension without creating more. Use birthdays or names with particular letters
- Pointing out role models if you can find any, such as a female garage mechanic, a female doctor or a male nurse.

## Care values in early years settings

- **Anti-discriminatory practice** – Not judging people because of their culture, race, religion, sexual identity, age, gender, health status, etc.
- **Confidentiality** – Service users have the right to say who should have access to personal data; care workers are responsible for respecting the service user's wishes
- **Culture, choice, personal identity and rights** – Each individual's personal beliefs and preferences – religious, cultural, political, ethical and sexual – must be respected
- The welfare of the child is paramount – you must always put the needs and wishes of the child first
- Keep the child safe and maintain a safe and healthy environment
- The child's learning and development must be promoted
- It is important to work in partnership with the child's parents and/or family

* It is important also that you work with other professionals in the best interest of the child – the contribution of others to the child's development must be valued
* As a professional you must always reflect upon your work so as to develop your skills.

### Protecting people at work

Most establishments have equal opportunities policies and codes of practice for dealing with racist remarks, attitudes or actions. Make sure you know who to report to if you see or hear anything you regard as racist. If matters are dealt with promptly it is less likely that feelings will run high and escalate into violence.

If situations of violence do break out because of racism then obviously this is a matter for the police and the courts.

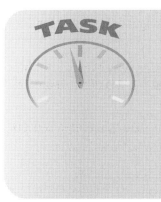

### TASK

### Recognise the diversity of service users

Write a detailed account to show how diversity is fostered in a care setting. You should show how equality could be fostered in the particular setting. You will also need to give detailed information about anti-discriminatory practice and the basis of discrimination, identify the different types of discrimination and give examples to show the different effects (physical, psychological and social) that discrimination can have on service users.

 **AO4** ## Recognise how to maintain confidentiality

Confidentiality is a principle common to all health, social care and early years services. Before any information you have gained is shared with other people the service user's permission must be obtained. If the reasons why you want to share the information are made clear to the service user, then consent is more likely to be given.

There are two levels of confidentiality.

On the first level, there are many things you need never speak about to anyone. If it is your task to help an older man who has wet himself to change his trousers, you do the task and say nothing. It is unprofessional to moan on the bus about what a fuss it was. How would you feel if it was your father, or indeed have you never been in an embarrassing situation yourself?

On the second level, when someone is discussing an issue with you, you may need to warn them that if they tell you that a crime has been committed or that the rules of the establishment you are in have been broken, then you will have to pass the information on. For example, if someone in a hostel is about to tell you that they sniff glue, you must make it clear to them that you will need to speak to someone more senior about it. If they have already told you, the same rule applies.

There are times when service user confidentiality has to be limited:

- If the service user is a danger to themselves or others
- If they are unconscious and cannot give information about their medical history
- If they are about to commit or have committed a crime
- If a court of law (not the police) requests information
- If abuse has taken place or is about to take place.

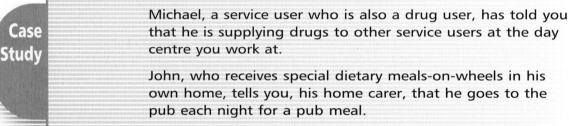

**Case Study**

Michael, a service user who is also a drug user, has told you that he is supplying drugs to other service users at the day centre you work at.

John, who receives special dietary meals-on-wheels in his own home, tells you, his home carer, that he goes to the pub each night for a pub meal.

Siobhan, who is a child in your class, tells you that 'Mummy's boyfriend' has hit her.

*Would you break confidentially in any of these situations? If you think you would, why?*

*What is confidential and what is not?*

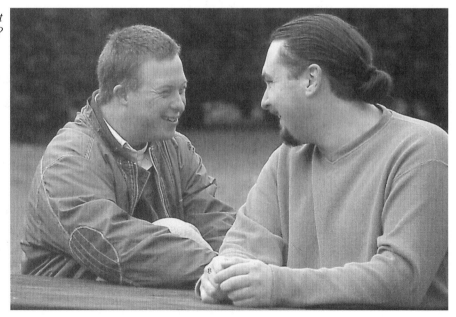

## Legislation

One of the key rights of service users is to be involved in how information about themselves can be kept out of official records and how it may be shared and used. Much good practice relating to confidentiality involves good interactive skills. For the purposes of Unit One, you will need to know how issues of confidentiality are governed in the care professions.

There are laws relating to confidentiality: the most relevant are the Data Protection Act 1984 and the 1995 European Directive on Data Protection, which came into force in October 1998. Although the Data Protection Act only covers computerised records, it is considered good practice also to apply it to both written (paper-based) and spoken communication. In any event, the European Directive extended many aspects of the Data Protection Act to paper-based records. Most healthcare, care and early years services must register with the Data Protection Registrar, who enforces the Act.

The Access to Medical Records Act 1988 and the Access to Health Records Act 1990 permit service users to have access to their own medical records and also allow them to prevent information from being passed on to other people without their consent.

## Policies/complaints procedures

Care agencies also have their own policies about confidentiality, which are often enforceable through their employees' contracts of employment. There are also professional codes of conduct enforced by professional associations such as the General Medical Council (for doctors) and the United Kingdom Central Council for Nursing, Midwifery and Health Visiting.

Service users may, of course, always use the complaints procedures that all care services have in place.

Service users must be told:

- Why information needs to be collected – this should be explained to the service user first, and their agreement obtained
- That written notes will be made of the discussion and that these notes will be written up and checked with the service user for accuracy before being entered into any official files
- How decisions are reached about the information that will be recorded and who will have access to the case file.

It is important in all matters of confidentiality that the service user understands fully how personal information will be dealt with, and that all file entries are checked with them for accuracy. The care worker should be sure that the service user does understand this.

## Organisation requirements, policies, procedures, recording, storage and security

An organisation that has any kind of information on service users must have a written policy on procedures for recording information and for storing it securely. Information must be in a secure room or secure cabinet and be only available to named persons. Much information today is stored on computers and these must be protected by secure passwords so that only certain people have access to the records.

## Support from line managers

If someone trusts you sufficiently to talk to you deeply about themselves or their problems, then this trust should never be broken. It is demeaning to the other person if you chat about them openly. It would also be very distressing to anyone who knew the other person. If you need help yourself because of what the service user has told you, then you must go to your supervisor in private.

## Organisation policies

This section of the unit will examine the many ways in which care organisations may promote equality and rights. Generally, this will be achieved through both policies and procedures.

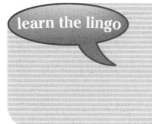

**learn the lingo**

**Policies** explain in broad terms what the organisation is trying to achieve. **Procedures** set out in detail how work within the organisation must be conducted. A procedure will state the ways in which decisions will be made, by whom and within what time-scale.

There are many things to consider when developing policies and procedures relating to equality and rights in care services. There often has to be a balance between bureaucratic mechanisms and professional judgements. Firm but sensitive handling is often required, and this is a very skilled area of work. As we have seen, it is made even more complex by the fact that sometimes the service itself must make decisions that involve service users' rights.

### Unacceptable risks for the service user

As we have noted, many of the criteria for the restriction of choice and rights are established in law. The removal of an individual's rights and choice is a legal and formal decision, often taken only by professionals issued with the legal authority to do so. When such decisions are made, they will be incorporated into the care plan for the service user, and all care workers will be made aware of their responsibilities. When a service user's rights or wishes are denied, for whatever reason, this should be explained appropriately to the service user and recorded in a file or reported to the appropriate worker. Such an action can never be casual or informal.

Sometimes a service user's wishes may be denied because of the impact they may have on others. All of us are sometimes restricted in our activities in relation to others. We may not be racist, obscene or physically belligerent.

The same applies to users of health and social care services, and this becomes particularly important in communal situations such as residential homes and hospitals.

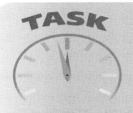

**TASK**

### Recognise how to maintain confidentiality

Confidentiality is a very important aspect of a carer's work with service users and it is important that you should have a good level of understanding of the legislation and policies that help to maintain confidentiality in care settings.

Choose two pieces of legislation (e.g. the Data Protection Act 1984, the Access to Personal Files Act 1987, the Access to Medical Records Act 1988) and two policies and show how these help to maintain confidentiality in a care setting. Use a wide range of examples to show how confidentiality is maintained; these should include oral, written and computerised information.

Confidentiality is an important care value but there are a number of situations when disclosure of certain information is necessary. Give examples of when information should be shared with others and give reasons why the sharing of confidential information may be necessary in these situations

**AO5** ## Review how legislation and policies help to maintain quality care

### Key legislation

#### Legislation supporting non-discriminatory practice

Some legislation makes it illegal to treat individuals unfairly because of prejudice or stereotyping, or seeks to promote the interests of groups who are vulnerable to discrimination. The following legislation is all relevant.

**The Sexual Offences Act 1967** legalised consenting sexual activity between men in private, provided that both parties were over 21 years of age (in England and Wales). Recently, this has been controversially lowered to 18 years of age, but it still does not provide equality for homosexuals with heterosexuals, for whom the age of consent is 16 years.

**The Chronically Sick and Disabled Persons Act 1970** suggested a range of services to be made available to disabled and ill people, including the provision of telephones and functional adaptations to their homes. This Act only set out guidelines. It instructed local authorities to provide services for disabled people and legislated (made it law) that new public buildings must provide access for disabled people.

The services that the Act recommended should be available to disabled people include:

- Home care workers (home helps)
- Meals-on-wheels
- Adaptations to homes
- Telephones
- Aids to daily living
- Occupation at home and at centres
- Outings
- Provision of transport.

The Act also stated that local authorities had to know how many disabled people there were in their area.

**The Equal Pay Act 1975** made it unlawful to discriminate between men and women doing the same jobs, in terms of their pay and conditions. Despite this landmark piece of legislation, statistical evidence shows that women still face discrimination in employment and pay. In addition, occupations such as nursing, which are perceived (wrongly!) as being largely women's work, are still extremely low-paid. The Act was amended in 1983 to comply with the (then) EC law.

**The Sex Discrimination Act 1975 and 1986** set out the rights of all individuals in issues regarding gender. The Act made it illegal to discriminate on the grounds of gender or marital status in education and employment. It also allowed for positive action in some cases, where being of a particular sex may be regarded as a genuine occupational requirement for a job. This Act set up the Equal Opportunities Commission to monitor and provide advice on promoting sexual equality.

**The Race Relations Act 1976** made it illegal to discriminate on the grounds of race, colour, ethnic origin or nationality. This Act is monitored by the Commission for Racial Equality, which the Act established and to which complaints may be brought. Specific responsibilities are placed on local authorities, which have a duty to eliminate racial discrimination and to promote equality. Nevertheless, racial discrimination still pervades British society.

The Act outlines:

- **Direct discrimination** – treating a person less favourably on the grounds of race
- **Indirect discrimination** – applying criteria that work to the disadvantage of one race over another.

It also makes victimisation illegal – it is illegal to treat somebody unfairly for being involved in making a complaint about discrimination.

The Race Relations (Amendment) Act 2000:

- Extends protection by increasing the responsibilities of public authorities
- Makes police Chief Constables liable for any discrimination by their officers
- Places new responsibilities on small employers to not discriminate
- Makes it illegal for people who manage property to discriminate when selling, letting or managing property.

**The Education (Handicapped Children) Act 1980** intended to fit children with special educational needs into mainstream education where possible. This responsibility is placed on local authorities. Children with disabilities are to be assessed and 'statemented'. The 'statement' defines the specific educational needs of the child, which the local authority is to meet through mainstream provision.

**The Mental Health Act 1983** safeguarded the rights of patients compulsorily admitted to hospital under the Act. It ensured that patients are made aware of their rights, and increased the role of the 'approved' social worker, in recognition of the importance of balancing medical and social factors in psychiatric illness. The Act is monitored by the Mental Health Act Commission.

**The Disabled Persons Act 1981 and 1986** increased the rights of disabled people by establishing the necessity for them to be informed about provision and consulted about their requirements. There are four main rights:

- Assessment of need is required by the local authority
- Resources must be provided, appropriate to the individual, that help the person to live as independently as possible
- Representation is a right of all disabled people. (Where the ability to express one's own needs is limited, representation may be made by another person or an advocate)
- Monitoring and review are necessary to reflect the changing needs of individuals with disabilities.

The Act intended to involve disabled people and their carers fully. However, its effectiveness nationally has been limited, as it only set out guidelines and suggestions. No responsibilities were imposed on either the National Health Service or local authorities. Recent attempts to improve the rights of people with disabilities have been systematically defeated and discouraged by the government.

**The Disabled Persons Act 1988** obliged companies employing more than 20 people to have 3% of their staff made up of disabled people.

**The National Health Service and Community Care Act 1990** ensured that individuals in need of care are appropriately assessed and have rights of complaint. The Act allows for service purchasing by authorities and sets out responsibilities for all care agencies, both statutory and independent, to work together. It had been anticipated that an individual's needs and preferences could be better met through these provisions. However, lack of money and competition among agencies for funds have rendered the Act far less effective than it might have been. In addition, the Act restricted real choice for those individuals who could not wholly finance their own care.

**The Criminal Justice Act 1992** places a duty on those administering the criminal justice system to avoid discrimination on the grounds of race or gender. In addition, its new sentencing structure was meant to provide more alternatives to prison. Since the introduction of the Act, however, prisons have been pushed beyond their capacity.

**The Fair Employment Act 1989** covers the area of religious discrimination in Northern Ireland. There is as yet (2003) no legislation relating to religious discrimination in England and Wales.

**The Employment Protection Act 1978** was concerned with rights to guarantee pay, medical suspension, time off work, maternity rights, sick pay and access to computerised data. Trade unions could be recognised at the discretion of the employer. Recognised unions can insist on equal opportunities policies and analysis of data to indicate how many black and white, male and female, disabled and non-disabled workers are employed by the company.

Although legislation or laws exist, discrimination continues because it takes a long time to change people's attitudes and ways of thinking. We can only challenge bad practice when we see it and try to promote as much good practice as possible.

**The Disability Discrimination Act 1995** introduced new rights for people with disabilities in employment, transport, education and access to goods and services. Employers with 20 or more employees are required to treat people with a disability no less favourably than any other employee. Employers have to provide facilities to allow people with disabilities to be employed in the workplace.

## Human Rights legislation

The Council of Europe is also active in enhancing Europe's cultural heritage in all its diversity. It acts as a forum for examining a whole range of social problems, such as social exclusion, intolerance, the integration of migrants, the threat to private life posed by new technology, bioethical issues, terrorism, drug trafficking and criminal activities.

The Council of Europe has established the European Convention on Human Rights, which is designed to protect individuals' fundamental rights and freedoms. The Council has set up a judicial procedure that is unique in the world and allows individuals to bring actions against governments if they consider that they are the victims of a violation of the Convention.

The existing two-level system, in which complaints are dealt with first by the European Commission and then by the European Court of Human Rights, will be replaced by a single and permanent Court; this will be more rapid and effective and complainants will have direct access to the Court.

### The Human Rights Act 1999

The Human Rights Act came into force on 2 October 2000. It gives every person clear legal rights based on the European Convention on Human Rights. Those rights can be enforced in UK courts and tribunals against public authorities – and against private bodies that are carrying out public functions.

For public authorities, the Act makes it a legal duty to act compatibly with the Convention rights. If a person's rights are harmed, s/he can take the public authority to court in the UK.

What is a public authority? The Act doesn't give a precise definition. But 'public authority' covers all central and local government bodies, the courts, the police and all government agencies. It also covers private bodies whose work includes government-type functions. Wherever you work in health or social care, if you are carrying out some public service on behalf of the State the chances are that you are covered by the Human Rights Act for at least some of your work. The Act applies to the care and health services as well as to housing and education provision.

The Human Rights Act ensures that the government's responsibilities for human rights can be met even when a private body carries out a public function such as providing meals-on-wheels or residential care, because it is carrying out a 'public function'. The following types of organisation are covered by the Act:

- Privatised utilities that exercise public functions (water authorities, electricity supply authorities)
- Regulatory bodies and professional associations in their regulatory

capacities such as the British Association of Social Workers, the Royal College of Nursing, the British Medical Association, the Central Council for Nursing, Midwifery and Health Visiting.

- Some charities and other voluntary organisations that carry out public functions for or instead of central or local authorities – such functions could include running a residential home
- Private or independent schools
- Bodies that are legally public corporations (organisations that provide services such as rail or bus companies).

The Act deliberately does not explain the meaning of 'public authority' or 'public function' in detail. It is for the courts to interpret the Act and to decide what are 'public authorities' and 'public functions' and what are not.

What rights does the Act cover? Some of the most important rights are listed below:

- **Article 3** – The right to freedom from inhuman or degrading treatment, which could be relevant to conditions in a residential care facility
- **Article 6** – The right to a fair hearing, not just in criminal trials but also in things like planning enforcement procedures or housing benefit review boards
- **Article 8** – The right to respect for private and family life, which could be relevant to issues involving respect for someone's private information or privacy in a residential care facility
- **Article 9** – The right to freedom of thought, conscience and religion; for example, there could be situations where someone's religious beliefs require or prevent him/her from doing something, like wearing particular clothes or working on a holy day.

### Religion and Sexual Orientation Amendment Regulations

New equality legislation outlawing discrimination in employment and vocational training on grounds of religion or belief, and on grounds of sexual orientation, will come into force in December 2003.

The introduction of this legislation, the Employment Equality (Religion or Belief) Regulations 2003 and The Employment Equality (Sexual Orientation) Regulations 2003, is a major step towards tackling unfair discrimination and will also outlaw discrimination and harassment on grounds of religion or belief and sexual orientation by trustees and managers of occupational pension schemes.

## Mission statements

A mission statement is an outline of what the service hopes to do.

## Mission statement

The aim of the Elms Nursing Home is to provide a residential and nursing service of the highest quality for the service users and staff within the resources available.

It is our objective to provide the service with high standards in care. Value for money is to be achieved at all times by the means and encouragement of a well trained and motivated workforce. We are committed towards the achievement of quality standards throughout the service, bringing job satisfaction to all employees.

Find out what the mission statement is for your college or school. The local Social Services department will also have a mission statement.

## Charters

In addition to legislation, there are a variety of government charters that indicate the rights and legitimate expectations of service users. These include the Citizen's Charter, which outlines what all users of public services have a right to expect. If services do not meet the required standards, the procedures for complaints are made clear.

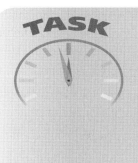

**TASK**

### Understand how legislation helps to maintain quality care in care settings

Choose three pieces of legislation and explain:

1. The purpose of each of the chosen pieces of legislation
2. How it is applied in care settings. Show how the legislation applies to service users and carers in the chosen care settings.

 **AO6**

## Conduct a survey to investigate how a care setting maintains quality care

You need to choose one aspect of care and carry out a survey to determine how the setting maintains quality.

For example you might wish to look at the quality of the **individual care plans** used by the setting. You could use the answers to the following questions to determine the quality of care offered. You could ask if:

- A comprehensive assessment is drawn up with each service user that provides the basis for the care to be delivered
- The plan sets out in detail the action that must be taken by care staff to ensure that all aspects of the health, personal and social care needs of the service user are met

- The plan meets relevant clinical guidelines produced by the professional bodies concerned with the care of older people and includes a risk assessment, with particular attention to prevention of falls?

- The plan is reviewed by care staff in the home at least once a month, updated to reflect changing needs and current objectives for health and personal care, and actioned

- The plan is drawn up with the involvement of the service user, recorded in a style accessible to them and agreed with and signed by them whenever they are capable of doing so.

You might instead survey how the setting provides for **the privacy and dignity of the service user**. You could use the answers to the following questions to determine the quality of privacy offered. You could ask if:

- The arrangements for health and personal care ensure that service user's privacy and dignity are respected at all times in situations such as:

  - personal care-giving, bathing, washing, using the toilet or commode

  - consultation with, and examination by, health and social care professionals such as nurses and doctors

  - consultation with legal and financial advisors

  - maintaining social contacts with relatives and friends

  - when carers are entering bedrooms, toilets and bathrooms

  - following death

- Service users have easy access to a telephone for use in private and receive their mail unopened

- Service users wear their own clothes at all times

- All staff use the term of address preferred by the service user

- All staff are instructed during induction on how to treat service users with respect at all times

- Medical examination and treatment are provided in the service user's own room

- Where service users have chosen to share a room, screening is provided to ensure that their privacy is not compromised when personal care is being given or at any other time.

## Conducting and presenting a successful survey

You will need to carry out a survey to investigate how a selected care setting maintains quality care, presenting a detailed survey plan that sequences tasks and reasons for those tasks. To gain a pass you can ask your teacher or tutor for help but if you wish to gain a merit or distinction you must carry out the survey without supervision. You must also remember when carrying out the survey to maintain confidentiality and to draw up a comprehensive questionnaire that covers in detail how a care setting fosters service users' rights, equality and diversity.

## Planning the survey

- Select the survey topic – what aspects of service users rights, equality and diversity are you going to survey?
- Decide on your approach, for example, observation or questionnaire
- Formulate your plan – how are you going to carry out the research, collect data, etc.?
- Carry out the project to collect the data and information
- Analyse and interpret the data
- Write up the survey.

## Information gathering for the survey

However you choose to collect your information and data, there are certain activities that are common:

- You must know where to locate the information and make arrangements to access it
- The information must be collected and recorded in a form suitable for analysis
- The information you gather must be relevant to your survey. A sample of services users' views on a quality matter collected on a Monday only would not give you enough data to generalise about all users or routines.

Record your information properly and in particular state the conditions under which you gathered the information.

## How can you record your information?

- **Log book** – This is the simplest method: the interviews, books read and information gathered can be recorded in a simple exercise book
- **Interview or survey notes** – This method is useful if you are carrying out open-ended interviews in which you are encouraging the people you are interviewing to express opinions or elaborate on a subject
- **On video** – Lightweight video cameras are excellent for recording information.

Before you decide what information to collect you should consider the following points:

- How long have you been given to carry out the survey?
- How available is the information?
- How accessible is the information?

- Can you do all you want to do in the time given?
- Have you the skills to carry out the survey – do you need help from your tutor?

There are a number of reasons why you may experience difficulty in carrying out the survey. The first of these difficulties is selecting a suitable topic or field of study and the second difficulty is managing your time.

## Time management

Let us suppose that you are going to carry out a survey of parents' opinions of quality issues in local day nursery.

You can see from the list of activities in Table 1.1 that for a simple survey you need to think in terms of at least 8 weeks. Planning your time is a very important aspect of carrying out surveys.

*Table 1.1 A time plan*

| Activity description | Estimated duration in weeks |
|---|---|
| Discuss with tutor | 1 |
| Discuss with nursery | 1 |
| Produce first draft of questionnaire | 1 |
| Discuss with tutor and finalise questionnaire | 1 |
| Administer questionnaire | 2 |
| Analyse results | 1 |
| Write up report | 1 |
| Total | 9 |

## How to gather information for the survey

Everybody observes other people at work or in other social situations. There is an important difference, however, between the observations of the student carrying out a survey and someone observing drinkers in a pub. Why is this? Because you must organise and analyse your data in a logical, systematic and sensitive manner. The ordinary person relies primarily on memory but you will attempt to keep written descriptions of what you see. For this reason, you are forced to think of systematic ways to conduct your survey.

## Observation as a method of collecting information

One method you could use to find out about how people behave is to observe them. For example, if you wanted to find out how carers behave in the dining room of a day unit, how would you go about it?

You could get a part-time job in the unit, sit down with the residents, eat a meal with them and observe the carers' behaviour. Alternatively, you could visit the unit, sit apart from the carers and watch what they do.

The first method (**participant observation**) has a high degree of interaction and the second method (**non-participant observation**) a low degree of interaction. Which method do you think would yield the data likely to give the deepest insight into the behaviour of the diners?

*It takes practice and careful planning to observe and record*

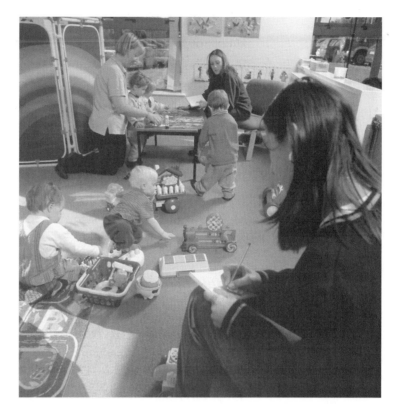

### Interviews and questionnaires as methods of collecting information

Instead of observing what people do, would you get more relevant information if you asked what they are doing? A questionnaire is simply a list of questions and provides a relatively fast, effective and cheap method of obtaining information.

A good questionnaire requires a lot of thought and planning. You must ask yourself:

- What questions am I going to ask?
- Who am I going to ask?
- How am I going to record the answers?
- What am I going to do with the results?

Before you construct a questionnaire you must carry out some background reading and research into the subject of quality practice. This will give you some ideas of the questions that should be asked. You should read books, journals and leaflets to gain some general ideas about your survey.

Read the sample questions in the next section and rewrite each question so as to eliminate the flaws.

### Leading questions

These questions encourage the respondent to say 'Yes'. Therefore, these questions are biased.

- Do you think that the establishment should allow you to go to bed whenever you want?
- Don't you agree than the food is very good?

### Questions that presume

These questions presume that the respondent has done the actions defined in the question.

- When did the carers last involve you in making decisions about meals?
- How many cups of coffee have you had?

### Double-barrelled questions

These are questions that ask more than one thing at once.

- Do you think that the centre should spend less money on the garden and more on the dining room?

### Why carry out an unstructured interview?

The least structured form of interviewing is the **unstructured** or **non-directive** interview. Respondents are given no direction by the interviewer. They are encouraged to relate their experience and to reveal their opinions and attitudes as they see fit. This type of interview allows the respondents to express their opinions as well as answer the questions. They can let you know their real feelings about the subject of the question and therefore tend to answer more freely and fully.

Suppose that you have decided that your task is to discover as many specific kinds of conflict and tension between carers and service users as possible. You might arrange your interview questions as set out below. The four areas of possible conflict you want to explore are listed in question 3. The first two questions are to allow you to build up a rapport with the respondent.

1. What sort of problems do service users have in getting along with carers?

2. Have you had any disagreements with your carers?

3. Have you ever had any disagreement with carers about:

   a. What kind of food you like

   b. Having friend or relatives to visit

   c. Having your own GP attend you

   d. Smoking in the establishment?

What do you have to do to encourage people to complete and return the questionnaires? With all surveys there is the problem of people who may refuse to fill in your questionnaire or simply forget to do so. This makes your results less accurate. If your response rate is low, what can you do to improve it?

There are various methods, including the following, that you can use to improve the response rate:

- **Follow-up** – Write or telephone the people who have not responded
- **Length of questionnaire** – The shorter the better, as longer questionnaires tend not to be answered
- **Who gave out the questionnaire?** – If the respondents know you or the college, then they are likely to reply. However, where questions are of a confidential nature this may not be the case and in these instances you must stress **confidentiality** in your introductory letter
- **Introductory letter** – An appeal to the respondents to emphasise that they would be helping the interests of everyone seems to produce the best results
- **Method of return** – A stamped addressed envelope produces the best results. In an establishment, perhaps a box to leave the questionnaire in?
- **Format of the questionnaire** – A title that will arouse interest helps, as does an attractive and clear layout with plenty of room for hand-written answers.

### The self-administered questionnaire

The self- administered questionnaire has some positive advantages. People are more likely to express socially unacceptable attitudes and feelings when answering a questionnaire alone than when confronted by an interviewer. The greater the anonymity the more honest the response. Aside from the greater honesty that they may produce, self-administered questionnaires also have the advantage of giving a respondent more time to think.

This type of survey gives no opportunity for the respondent to probe beyond the answer. Therefore, the questions should be simple and straightforward, and be understood with the help of minimal, printed instructions.

# 2 Communicating with service users In care settings

## To complete this unit you will need to:

- Recognise how to encourage oral communication
- Investigate the range of skills used when communicating effectively
- Review how to communicate through effective listening
- Recognise how to apply the care values that underpin communicating with others
- Communicate effectively with service users
- Evaluate the range of communication skills used and plan for improvements.

 **AO1** Recognise how to encourage oral communication

One of the most likely reasons why you chose to do a course in Care is that you are interested in people. You may be the sort of person friends contact to talk over problems. You may have appreciated someone else listening to you to help you out. Your interest in people and in helping is a great advantage in health and social care situations when you may be expected to give service users support.

The fact that it is extremely difficult not to **communicate** shows how important communication is. At a fun level, see how long you can manage without communication – not talking to your student colleagues for example! On a more serious note, think how hard it is for those in solitary confinement. Our instinct is to communicate with others because relationships hinge on communication and without relationships living would be mere existence.

Why do you need to communicate with service users?

You communicate with service users to get information to meet their physical, social, emotional and intellectual needs.

To meet these needs you need to:

- Listen and respond to what people say to you
- Use good eye contact and keep smiling
- Be sincere, sympathetic and understanding
- Be kind, gentle and tactful
- Be willing to assist, but always allow the person to do as much as possible for themselves
- Encourage them to be as independent as possible
- Show empathy
- Know when to keep quiet
- Know how to 'read' and use non-verbal communication, such as facial expressions, use of eye contact and posture
- Know how to ask questions
- Respect people as individuals
- Listen to their point of view.

Communication is a two-way process. You need a person to send a communication (for instance, to speak) and a person to receive (listen) to have effective communication.

The whole process involves a person sending a message to another person. That person receiving the message (who has to understand it) then sends a message back (feedback) to the person who sent the original message (see below).

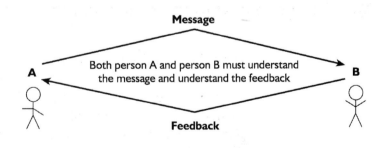

Communication is important because it helps us to:

- Live our lives practically
- Develop psychologically and intellectually
- Express ourselves emotionally
- Form relationships socially.

## Communication in health and social care

There are several types of communication or interaction important in health and social care. These include:

- **Language** – The use of words in making statements and asking questions, also known as verbal behaviour; the use of language includes how we emphasise words, and our tone of voice
- **Sensory contact** – This includes non-verbal behaviour such as body language, facial expression, distance from the other person and touching
- **Activity interaction** – This may consist of activities such as music, arts and crafts, drama and movement. Sometimes it is more effective to allow individuals to communicate through activity, and opportunities for this may be provided by, among others, occupational therapists.

All forms of effective interpersonal interaction require skill and training.

## Why is communication so important in health and social care?

Within health and social care, there are very specific reasons why communication is so important:

- Exchange of information between carer and service user
- So the carer can explain procedures
- So the carer can develop and promote relationships
- So the carer can negotiate (act as advocate) on behalf of and with the service user and empower them
- Promotion of interaction within groups.

### Exchange of information

Much of the work within health, social care and early years services requires information to be exchanged between workers and service users, between workers and workers, between workers and their organisation, and between organisations. For example, in order for an assessment to be made of the needs of an individual, some form of interview must occur.

The skills of the care worker will need to be good in order to extract and record reliable information.

### Explaining procedures

Clarity in communication is essential when explaining procedures, so that mistakes will not be made and also so that the service user has all the information necessary in order to make informed decisions. Procedures may include health treatments or investigations, how an assessment works, or even how complaints and appeals procedures work.

### Promoting relationships and offering support

Effective communication is also the core of the caring relationship – it communicates warmth, support, concern and approval. It is through effective communication that we can value people as individuals and make them feel empowered.

*Developing relationships*

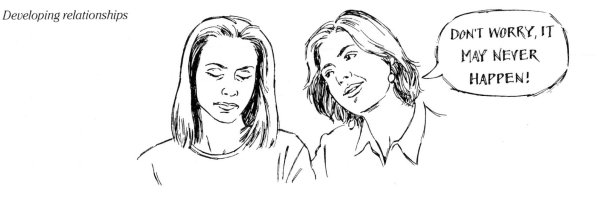

DON'T WORRY, IT MAY NEVER HAPPEN!

Care workers may have to negotiate and liaise with service users, family members, colleagues and other professionals. Care work requires effective communication with many different individuals who have an interest in the service being offered.

### Promotion of interaction between group members

Much care work (but not all!) requires working with a group or as part of a team. Care workers need to be able to make useful contributions to the group as well as to promote and support the contribution of others.

**Case Study**

Mrs Mackey is a very dependent 80-year-old lady who lives alone. She has a hearing disability and her eyesight is deteriorating. She receives meals-on-wheels every day.

*Why do you think it might be very important for the person who delivers meals to Mrs Mackey to have good communication skills?*

## Types of communication in care settings

Much communication and interaction in care services may be informal, e.g. getting to know service users and chatting with colleagues. While such interactions may seem natural and undemanding, the care worker will understand that the quality of service the service user receives and the environment within which the care worker works are highly dependent upon the quality of those interactions.

Other communications and interactions will be more formal, and these may include explaining decisions or procedures to service users and their families, assessing needs and confirming information, case conferences and staff meetings. In these situations, while clarity and accurate information are critical, the skills of the worker in being sensitive and caring are still paramount.

### Case Study

Mary is at a youth club with some of her friends. They decide to go as a group to a nearby club.

Sasha attends a local athletics club and is a member of the athletics team.

A case conference is held by a social care team to discuss a service user.

*Which of these situations is a formal group and which an informal group?*

## How effective communication helps to meet the needs of people

The effectiveness of your communication skills may depend on how far your approach meets the needs of the other person. For example, you will have to approach a 3-year-old child differently from the way you approach your tutor. Language, posture, pace and tone all need to be adapted to the other person.

*Formal relationships*

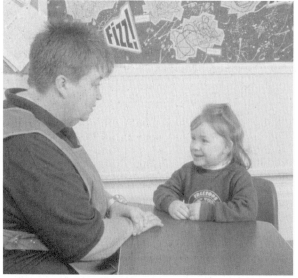

**Case Study**

*Mary is a home carer who is supporting Mrs Patel to live independently in her own home. Mary talks to Mrs Patel but does not take any notice of her answers. Mrs Patel expresses a wish to do some cooking but Mary thinks it would be best if she did it herself.*

*Has Mary's communication with Mrs Patel a positive or negative effect?*

*Do Mary's actions empower Mrs Patel?*

Care workers need to systematically develop their skills. Failure to do so may result in the service users becoming disempowered, feeling oppressed and losing their sense of self-worth. Care workers must be watchful and attentive in their interactions with others, recognising that interactions may have both positive and negative effects.

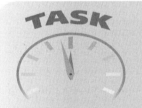

**TASK**

## Using interpersonal communication skills to empower service users

Choose a care setting in order to make notes on how effective communication is used by the service as a means of valuing people as individuals. You will need to make these notes over a period of time, and may also wish to ask questions of members of staff. You will also have to find out about how the service promotes confidentiality. There should be written policies on this.

1. Using specific examples from your notes, explain how the care service uses effective communication. For example, you may wish to describe how service users are given choices, are encouraged to express themselves and are listened to effectively. You must describe specific interactions and explain how the interaction respected and promoted the individual's dignity and self-esteem. Make sure you provide sufficient examples.
2. Describe how the organisation stores records and information about service users, and explain what rights service users or others may have to this information. You should refer to both legal requirements and organisational policies in order to discuss this. In what ways are service users made aware of their rights regarding confidentiality by the organisation?

## Why is communication important in developing relationships?

We tend to think of communication as speaking but there are many ways to communicate meaning or messages to others. It isn't just what we say that creates impressions, but also how we express the words, what we wear, how we stand, look, behave, listen and respond.

## What factors can influence communication?

Work on improving your listening skills and your questioning skills and be conscious of your body language, as these can all influence communication. Other physical or practical factors may influence your interaction with the other person – factors such as:

- Noise
- Interruptions from other people or from you
- Barriers such as desks or chairs
- The room temperature – it may be so cold or so hot that it is difficult to concentrate on the matter in hand
- Someone may be very tired or hungry – children and many adults find it hard to take in what is being said if they are tired, thirsty or hungry.

### Non-verbal communication

Non-verbal communication may be classed as a physical factor because it concerns the ways in which we use our bodies to communicate. We will discuss effective non-verbal communication later in this unit. Changes in the body language of others will provide reliable information as to whether they are angry, distressed, threatened, relaxed and happy, etc.

### The physical environment

The physical environment can also be a major factor in inhibiting effective communication. Interaction needs to occur in an appropriate environment.

If confidentiality is a concern, privacy will be important, so that the interaction will not be overheard. Too much noise or too many distractions can seriously inhibit the effectiveness of an interaction.

This aspect of the physical setting includes lighting, heating, levels and types of noise, odours and general cleanliness. These rather subtle variables can have a significant influence on the degree of comfort the service user experiences. Making service users comfortable is important. The physical ambience in the office, for example, should communicate that visitors are welcome; there should be good lighting, comfortable chairs and appropriate heating/temperature control.

## What other factors can inhibit effective communication?

We have discussed the fact that some forms of communication may be less effective than others. It is very important that you understand the differences between effective and non-effective communication. In this section, we shall explore the factors that make effective interaction difficult.

**Case Study**

Sandra is 26 years old and pregnant with her first child. She is a little worried about her health and wants some advice from the health visitor. She makes an appointment at her local health centre but when she arrives on time she is asked to wait; the receptionist gives no explanation. Sandra becomes distressed. The health visitor sees Sandra after about an hour and does not apologise or give an explanation for the delay. She rushes her into a cold office, leaves the door open and begins the conversation by saying 'Well ... '. She sits behind a large desk and Sandra has to sit in a low armchair.

*Identify the factors that inhibit effective communication between the staff of the health centre and Sandra.*

It is important that care workers are able to identify barriers to effective communication. Some of the barriers may be due to poor interpersonal skill development in the care worker. Other barriers may be due to the physical environment – poor building design, noise or lack of privacy.

Some service users may have special communication problems, such as:

- Deafness
- A speech impediment
- Memory difficulties.

There will be many occasions when the other person finds it difficult to talk because of emotional factors such as anger, shame or great sadness. Can you think of other emotional factors that might make interaction difficult?

Communication can be greatly enhanced by having a relaxed manner and communicating understanding, sincerity and warmth. However, care workers need to understand that, regardless of their own training, the most demanding situations will still arise. The professional caring relationship can be highly charged emotionally and it is important that you, the care worker, see the service user as the more important person in the relationship.

Many common emotional problems can arise in caring relationships that can make effective communication difficult. One such common problem is lack of self-awareness. Not all relationships will work or go smoothly. This is usually due to the care worker's lack of self-awareness in some areas.

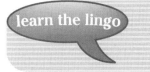

**Self-awareness** is understanding of how you are perceived by others and the impact you have on them.

In such situations regular supervision from a line manager is useful. Care workers have a professional obligation to strive continuously to develop their awareness and skills, and there is a responsibility on the part of the agency that employs them to ensure that this happens through the provision of supervision and continuing professional updating and development.

## Attitudes as barriers to effective communication

Some attitudes can create barriers, such as stereotyping, maintaining class distinctions or lacking respect for cultural and ethnic differences. Of course, not everyone speaks English, and an interpreter may be necessary. Another major barrier can be anger or distress, which effectively prevents open and honest communication. Identifying such barriers is the first step to overcoming them.

### What is stereotyping?

Unless you communicate with each person as an individual you are likely to make assumptions about them – that is, you make a judgement about them based on something you have seen or read. The judgement may be wrong but it affects your interaction with that person. The assumption grows to a stereotype – we make the person fit the image we have of them rather than accepting them for what they are. The stereotypes act as barriers to good communication.

Good carers try to be aware of the stereotypes they make, particularly when the person they are trying to communicate with is from a different social class, from a different ethnic background or of the opposite gender. Here are some examples of how we can easily misjudge people and get the wrong message.

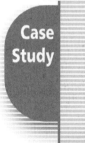

**Case Study**

John is a new care worker in a residential home for people with severe physical disabilities. He feels that all the residents are very dependent and that his role is to do everything for them. He does not see each user as an individual.

*Is John stereotyping all the users of the establishment?*

*How could John attempt to empower the service users?*

*How does his lack of awareness of the service users' disabilities affect John's ability to communicate effectively?*

### Gender

We are socialised into our gender roles from the minute we are born, by the colour of the blanket that is wrapped around us and the kind of card that is sent to greet us.

### Age

When did you last run a marathon? It is not only older people who do not normally take strenuous exercise. Negative stereotyping about age highlights sickness, dependency and not being able to be sociable. Others may see older people as retarded, slow or inefficient.

### Disability

Often assumptions are made about disabled people's abilities that are based on misunderstanding. Access and opportunities are very significant to disabled people. If they are denied access to a building or the opportunity to do a job then they cannot demonstrate the capabilities that they have.

The possible effects of discrimination are so pervasive and wide-ranging that it is impossible to explain or describe them in depth or with accuracy. Reading novels and poems, watching films or television programmes and listening to personal experiences can inform us about the possible effects of discrimination.

Everyone stereotypes to a certain extent. We make judgements about people in our minds so that we can interact with them. For example, if you met a young man wearing sports clothes you might assume that he enjoyed playing sport. If you met a teenage girl wearing trendy clothes you might assume that she liked listening to music and socialising. You might be very wrong in both cases, but the misjudgements are probably not damaging.

## How can culture and beliefs affect oral communication?

The problem may simply be one of language. The service user may not speak English very well. In such a situation, the care worker needs to find an interpreter.

**Case Study**

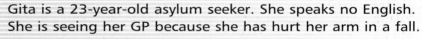

Gita is a 23-year-old asylum seeker. She speaks no English. She is seeing her GP because she has hurt her arm in a fall.

*What arrangements could the GP make to communicate effectively with Gita?*

## How can a lack of awareness of a service user's difficulties and disabilities affect communication?

The service user may be hearing-impaired, in which case the worker may have to use an alternative method of communicating, such as signing or writing, rather than talking to them. The service user's preferred method of communication should always be used.

A common problem is the use of technical jargon, particularly in medical settings. This should always be avoided, and the worker should attempt to communicate with the service user in ways that fit in with the service user's level of understanding and abilities.

The major point about communicating effectively as a care worker is that the responsibility for being understood always lies with the care worker.

## Using effective communication to empower service users

Interaction between care workers and service users should be empowering for the service user. Class, age, disability, gender and race may all contribute to individuals feeling that they lack power – that they are somehow 'unequal' to others. One of the goals of effective interaction is to establish a sense of partnership with service users. Skilful listening and questioning can help to empower service users.

Awareness of people's rights and preferences, helping people to talk about the past and listening attentively to their experiences can all help to empower.

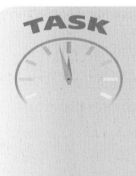

### TASK

### Recognise how to encourage oral communication

Communication is a very important aspect of care. To be successful in this assignment you will need to show the reasons why service users and care workers need to communicate.

1. You must show by giving examples that you have an understanding of factors that influence oral communication such as; – noise, lighting, ventilation, heating, space, etc. You also need to give examples to show that you appreciate how barriers such as distress, tiredness, inappropriate body language, etc. can inhibit oral communication with service users.
2. In order to communicate effectively we need to understand how certain key concepts can influence interactions. Explain and give examples of how stereotyping, labelling and lack of respect for service users can influence interactions. Give detailed examples to illustrate how cultural differences can influence oral communication between carers and service users.

Evidence for this assignment can be presented in writing or through the use of video and comment, or using records that your teacher may make.

Effective communication in health and care services can only ever be empowering when:

- It respects people's preferences and beliefs

- It promotes confidentiality and respects people's privacy
- It enables service users to express their views and be heard
- It promotes service users' rights
- It helps to develop individual identities in service users and supports personal development.

### The feeling of power

Sometimes care workers assume that, because they have the responsibility of caring for vulnerable people, they can make decisions for them. The powerlessness of the service user can provide a real sense of control on the part of the care worker. Think of how you felt when you last went to your GP or dentist. Would you do everything they asked you to do? Would you have questioned their diagnosis or medicine that the GP prescribed?

## AO2 Investigate the range of skills used when communicating effectively

Effective communication begins with the recognition that each person is different and unique.

Effective communication is essentially mutual understanding between the service user and the care worker. The responsibility for understanding the service user clearly lies with the care worker.

If care workers are not being understood, they must find another way of expressing themselves. If the service user is not being understood, the care worker must use a different technique of communication.

## What are the skills of interpersonal interaction?

There are five basic skills in enhancing an interaction with a service user:

- Questioning
- Self-disclosure and prompting
- Active listening
- Giving information
- Rapport.

Each of these involves both verbal and non-verbal skills.

### What is questioning?

Questioning is the seeking of information, clarification, views, feelings and thoughts. There are two basic types of questions: closed and open.

### What are closed questions?

Closed questions are questions that can be answered in one or two words, often 'Yes' or 'No.' 'What is your name?' 'How old are you?' 'Do you eat chips?' and 'What is your nationality?' are examples of closed questions. They are essential for ascertaining facts. Too many closed questions inhibit conversation.

## Open questions

Open questions are questions that require a more extended answer. For example, instead of asking a service user 'Do you eat pork?', the care worker might ask 'What sorts of foods do you like and dislike?' Such an open question feels more comfortable and allows service users to answer in their own way. The use of open questions communicates to the service user that the care worker is interested in the whole range of responses that the service user might make.

Open questions typically begin:

- How?
- Why?
- In what ways?
- What sort of?

It appears that the use of closed questions comes more naturally in our culture. In order to develop skill in open questioning, practice is required.

Although it is important to ask questions to clarify the situation or the problem, avoid asking too many. Otherwise, the service user will feel burdened and unable to talk freely.

Also avoid:

- **Saying to the service user, 'Don't worry – it really doesn't matter'.** This puts the problem down – it makes it seem small. To the service user the problem is big. S/he doesn't want to have it dismissed, s/he wants it talked through.
- **Telling the service user directly what to do.** There may be a course of action that is appropriate but you should try to arrange it so that the service user makes the decision him/herself.
- **Being loud and overbearing.** Obviously, if people have a hearing loss you have to speak up, but generally people appreciate a tone that's easy to listen to.
- **Rushing to get it over with.** You may be in a desperate hurry for a genuine reason and in this case you may have to ask to see the service user at another time. Usually, however, it is best to go at the pace of the person you are talking to.
- **Shifting the emphasis from the service user to yourself** and starting to recount your own experiences. Your service user doesn't want to hear about your problems.
- **Diagnosing 'what your problem is'.** By telling someone what their problem or need really is you are putting your own interpretation on it.

It is only the problem as you see it, and not necessarily the whole problem or the problem as it affects the other person's life. You are making a judgement about the service user and the situation they are in. You may have it all wrong.

## What is self-disclosure and prompting?

Self-disclosure is another means of enhancing a conversation when seeking information from the service user. It is often used in conjunction with questioning. The purpose of self-disclosure is to make service users more comfortable and forthcoming, by telling them something about yourself. This empathy with the service user helps to establish areas of common interest. Self-disclosure turns an interview into a conversation. Some examples of self-disclosure, used with an open question, might be:

'I don't like sweet desserts. What sorts of dessert do you like?'

'I broke my leg once and found using crutches very difficult. How are you managing with them?'

Self-disclosure is a type of prompting. Most of us prompt quite naturally, by nodding our heads or by saying 'Yeah' or 'I see' while the other person is talking. This sort of phrase, combined with an attentive gaze and raising of the eyebrows, are effective prompts. They tell the service user that we are expecting them to say more.

## What is active listening?

Questioning, prompting and self-disclosure are some of the ways in which we obtain information and enhance interaction. However, it is important that the care worker shows that the service user has been listened to and understood. This is called active listening. Active listening is a powerful way of optimising interactions.

There are two types of active listening:

● Paraphrasing
● Reflective listening.

Some of the ground rules are as follows:

● Avoid saying that you understand when you don't.
● Avoid jumping in with your own points of view.
● Use open questions.
● Pay attention to body language.

### What is paraphrasing?

Paraphrasing is a simple and effective way to test understanding. A paraphrase is a repetition or a summary of what the service user has said. It might begin with a phrase such as 'What you have been saying, if I've got it right, is . . .' and then repeating or summing up what the service user has said. Importantly, it communicates to the service user that the care worker has been listening and trying to understand.

### What is reflective listening

Reflective listening is less concerned with the summarising of facts and more involved with understanding the emotions and feelings that are being communicated by the service user. All interactions between people communicate only three basic things:

- Emotions and feelings
- Needs and wants
- Facts or opinions.

In reflective listening, the listener sorts out the information received from the other person into these categories, and responds only in the order above. Emotions and feelings are the first and most important aspect to respond to, using emotion and feeling words. Some examples of feeling words are:

| | |
|---|---|
| Happy | Angry |
| Worried | Frustrated |
| Sad | Frightened |
| Excited | Depressed |
| Concerned | Disappointed. |

How many more can you think of? Feeling words are important for identifying the emotions of those with whom we converse.

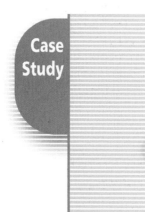

**Mr Wilkinson:** Mike usually helps me with my bath. He will be here in an hour. Can you help me now instead?

**Care worker:** You seem worried about Mike giving you your bath.

*Mr Wilkinson might feel inclined to discuss what is worrying him because the care worker has been able to label his emotion for him. If the care worker is mistaken, and Mr Wilkinson is not worried, he has an opportunity to correct the care worker's mistaken perception.*

Essentially, in reflective listening we are saying that how people feel is often more important than the facts or details of the situation.

## Communication with children

A feeling misread can give rise to many more incorrect responses. Reflective listening is one of the major skills of working with children.

**Fiona (aged 8)**: The teacher caught me messing around and kept me in during playtime.

**Care worker**: You must have felt embarrassed in front of your friends.

*The care worker invites Fiona to talk about what happened at school by suggesting that she might have felt embarrassed. To have been condemnatory of Fiona would have shut her up.*

Children need to have their feelings acknowledged. Much of our interaction with children is directive, prescriptive and factually based.

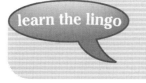

**Directive** means something that guides or tells. **Prescriptive** means something that lays down rules.

Telling a child that you can see when s/he is upset, happy or worried works wonders. Because you have acknowledged the child's feelings, the child is likely to talk more. Perhaps it is because we often do not use reflective listening with children that many children grow up without learning this important skill themselves.

*You are a worker in a reception class and a parent has just had to drop off her child, Sara, in a hurry to make another appointment. Sara is upset because her parent usually stays for about five minutes settling her in to the class.*

*How would you acknowledge Sara's feelings?*

## Behaviour that fails to value people

Carers must be very careful that they do not intentionally or unintentionally use behaviour that fails to value a service user. Talking about them, patronising them, shouting at them and not respecting their wishes are all unacceptable behaviour.

Any unacceptable behaviour makes service users feel that they are not respected and can lead to a lowering of their self esteem.

### The role of non-verbal behaviour and body language in communication

What we have been looking at up to this point is **verbal communication**.

Can we communicate without using words? A large part of communication is actually carried out without speaking – 'non-verbally' – we call this **non-verbal communication** or **body language**. In care settings this type of communication is very important.

How many kinds of non-verbal communication (body language) can you think of?

*Body language*

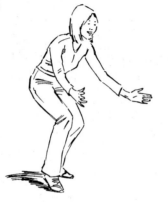

Communication skills depend not only on verbal skills but also on non-verbal skills and body language. We converse with our whole body, including facial expressions, eyes, gestures, physical distance and skin tone. Although we read body signals all the time, it takes considerable practice and skill to do this consciously. However, the non-verbal aspects of communication provide valuable clues about how an interaction is progressing and about the feelings of the other person.

### *Facial expression*

Our faces communicate complex and subtle messages. A smiling and alert face strongly attracts. A forlorn and helpless face arouses sympathy and concern.

### *Smiling*

One of the most significant signs is a smile. Smiling shows warmth and openness, which makes for positive interaction.

A tense and grumpy face sends out messages to stay away. A long, silent gaze with raised eyebrows evokes speech in the other person. We use our eyes to continue speech and to obtain feedback. We end conversations by looking away. People look more at the person they talk to when they like them, and also look more at the other person when they are listening than when they are talking.

### Eye contact

This is one of the most direct ways of communicating. Many of you will have received or made romantic intentions clear without speaking a word!

Where you focus your eyes makes a difference to the interaction, or two-way talk, you achieve. The length of your gaze also makes a difference. It is not a good idea to stare the service user out but it is necessary to look at the service user so that they know they have your attention.

*The length of your gaze also makes a difference*

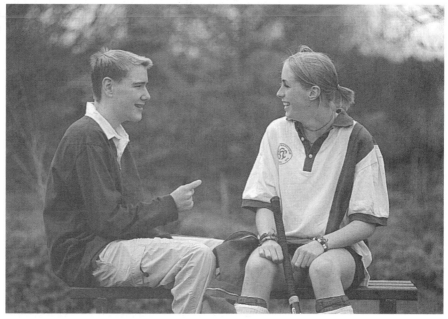

### Positive positioning

All of us require personal space. The amount that we require is partly determined by culture as well as by personal preference. The amount of personal space used in an interaction is important in relation to intimacy and dominance. The closer the person gets, the more intimate or dominant they wish to be. We all like to be in control of our personal space and the situations in which we wish to be close (intimate) with someone. For example, in a doctor's waiting room, people keep their distance from one another, unless numbers force them to sit close together. To sit down right next to another person in an otherwise empty waiting room would make that person extremely uncomfortable.

Have you ever noticed how people stand a safe distance apart when they don't know each other? Have you ever felt uncomfortable when somebody you don't know has edged on to your side of the seat on a train or on a bus? Some people actually stand very close to you when they talk and this makes you feel uneasy.

Everyone has his or her own '**personal space**'. This is the space that they need for themselves where only those they know well can enter. When people are compelled to be unusually near to each other for some reason, in a railway carriage for example, they often adopt little mechanisms to avoid catching the eye of the person near them, such as staring out of the window or concentrating on the newspaper or a book.

*Personal space differs according to circumstances*

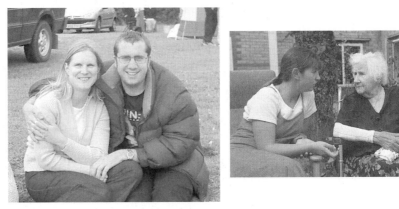

Body contact is another area of intimacy. Here also the British use less physical contact than many other cultures. Touching is an area of great importance in care; some service users welcome physical contact while others do not. It is a good idea to be guided by the way the service user him/herself uses touch. If service users are physically expressive, they may not mind you mirroring their use of touch. However, if a service user appears not to use touch, it is better to interact with them in the same way.

## Case Study

Mrs Hector is a 90-year-old service user in a residential home. She has just received a letter saying that a very good friend had died.

*How would you communicate to Mrs Hector that you understand the feelings she is experiencing? Would you use verbal communication or non-verbal communication skills?*

## Gestures and body postures

### Gestures

How do we use our hands in communication? Drumming our fingers implies impatience, as might jangling keys in pockets or twiddling thumbs. Sometimes people use their hands to cover their faces and this may imply they have something to hide – they are being defensive.

*Posture is very important*

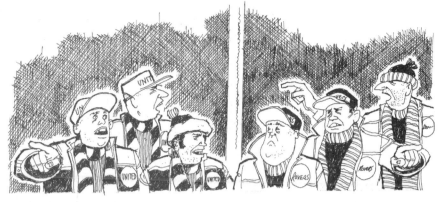

### Touch

This is a very tricky aspect of non-verbal communication and needs some confidence. Occasionally, a hand on someone's shoulder or arm can be very reassuring, and with children giving a hug after a bad fall can be a spontaneous response to a distressed child.

The issue of physical contact can easily be misunderstood or misrepresented if an incident is retold in the wrong way. This is particularly true if different genders are involved, for example in the case of a male nursery nurse working with children. In these circumstances your actions must always be above any criticism. Other staff must be involved.

*Appropriate touching*

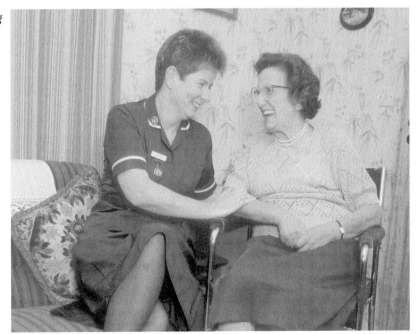

## Makaton

Makaton is a method of communicating used mostly with service users with a learning disability. Many of the signs used in Makaton are used in

British sign language. Makaton uses signs and facial expressions to communicate. Speech is always used with the signs.

Signs and symbols give extra information which can be seen. Signs/gestures are easier to learn than spoken words. This makes sense. Makaton can help if a child has difficulties with understanding and speaking. Through Makaton, the child is able to develop important communication skills.

The following figure shows examples of some signs used in communicating with Makaton.

*Makaton signs: a system used by many children and adults who have communication difficulties*

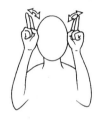
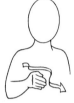
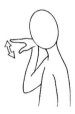

boy
brush right index
finger pointing
left across chin

rabbit
Palm forward 'N'
hands, held at either
side of head, bend
several times to
indicate ears

fish
Right flat hand
waggles forward
like a fish
swimming

bird
Index finger and
thumb open and
close in front of
mouth like a beak

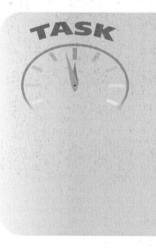

## Investigate the range of skills used when communicating effectively

Oral skills are important when communicating with service users.

1. Describe four oral skills you would use when communicating with a service user and explain why and in what situation you would use each skill. Also show how body language can contribute to effective communication.
2. Describe three example of behaviour that would show that the carer was failing to value the service user and the possible effect of this failure on the service user.

**AO3**  ## Review how to communicate through effective listening

A good listener hears the content of what the speaker says and the intent – what the person means.

Listen actively. Get ready to listen. Make the shift from speaker to listener a complete one.

Think whether your body language conveys messages like 'Yes, I am

*Think of our interactions*

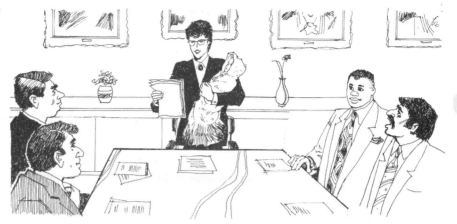

listening. I want to hear what you say' or 'No, I'm eager to leave. I'm not interested'. Sitting beside the person you are talking to without distractions or 'blocks' such as a desk separating you makes the difference between good and poor communication patterns. Stretching back in your chair away from the person sends messages of distance and carelessness, while leaning forward, nodding, saying 'Yes' or making quiet utterances such as 'Mm' makes the service user more aware of your interest.

*Barrier to effective communication*

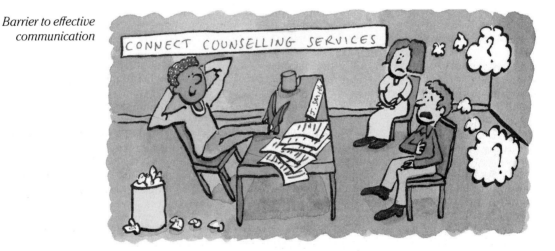

You must really focus and try to remember what the person has said.

A key to understanding emotions is to describe them! It can be helpful to suggest a particular word to the person that might describe their feelings. This means building up your language skills. Sometimes you need to put what has been said into your own words.

## How we can use effective listening to help people?

As you listen actively and try to reflect back to the person their feelings and what they say, you will gradually move towards empathy. That is, you will be able to put yourself in the other person's position. You need to empathise in order to be able to help the person effectively.

Silence is golden . . . .

We have so far emphasised the importance of listening, but sometimes people may just need a little space to be quiet. They need moments to pause, to regain themselves, to think of the words they need. It is not always easy to express feelings because it may be painful or embarrassing and there may be silence. Try to use the silence; try not to be tense about it. Even skilled carers can find silences difficult to handle. You may eventually be able to question gently.

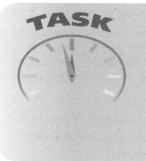

## TASK

### Effective listening

Oral skills and behaviour are important factors in communicating, as is the use of listening skills.

Explain four factors that aid effective listening and give examples of how these could contribute to effective listening when communicating with service users.

## AO4 Recognise how to apply the care values that underpin communicating with others

### Personal values and attitudes

Much of our interpersonal interaction is guided by our personal values and attitudes. What we think is right and true affects the way we behave. Many of the ideas and assumptions we have are based on what we were told as children and later on what we have seen and heard on television or read about. We hinted at this in Unit 1 when discussing stereotypes and discrimination. Sometimes our own prejudices or personal fears and values are more subtle but are still significant in affecting how we relate to people.

### Care values

The care **values** are principles, standards or qualities considered worthwhile or desirable by the care profession. An individual's attitudes and values can be observed in their behaviour. Although it is difficult to change attitudes, and hence values, some vocations, such as health and social care, require a great deal of attention to be paid to them.

All health and care workers must ensure that their attitudes and values do not influence their own behaviour.

Three care values are:

- **Anti-discriminatory practice** – Not judging people because of their culture, race, religion, sexual identity, age, gender, health status, etc.
- **Confidentiality** – Service users have the right to say who should have access to personal data – care workers are responsible for respecting the wishes of the service user
- **Individual rights and choice, personal beliefs and identity** – Each individual's own personal beliefs and preferences – religious, cultural, political, ethical and sexual – must be respected.

## Care values in early years settings

- **Anti-discriminatory practice** – Not judging people because of their culture, race, religion, sexual identity, age, gender, health status, etc.
- **Confidentiality** – Service users have the right to say who should have access to personal data; care workers are responsible for respecting the service user's wishes
- **Culture, choice, personal identity and rights** – Each individual's personal beliefs and preferences – religious, cultural, political, ethical and sexual – must be respected
- The welfare of the child is paramount – you must always put the needs and wishes of the child first
- Keep the child safe and maintain a safe and healthy environment
- The child's learning and development must be promoted
- It is important to work in partnership with the child's parents and/or family
- It is important also that you work with other professionals in the best interest of the child – the contribution of others to the child's development must be valued
- As a professional you must always reflect upon your work so as to develop your skills.

### *Equality for all individuals*

The intention of having care values is to create equality for all individuals. Most professional carers are employed by agencies that have considerable power and that also have responsibilities in law to others besides service users. While we emphasise the therapeutic, supportive and counselling roles of care workers, they are also responsible to the agency they work for. A care worker may possess more power, through position, than their service user. To counteract these processes the care worker should:

- Identify and question his/her own values and prejudices, and their implications for practice
- Respect and value uniqueness and diversity, and recognise and build on strengths

- Promote people's rights to choice, privacy, confidentiality and protection while recognising and addressing the complexities of competing rights and demands

- Assist people to increase control of, and improve the quality of, their lives while recognising that control of behaviour will be required at times in order to protect people from harm

- Identify, analyse and take action to counter discrimination, racism, disadvantage, inequality and injustice, using strategies appropriate to the situation

- Practise in a manner that does not stigmatise or disadvantage individuals, groups or communities.

### Confidentiality

This is a principle common to all health, social care and early years services. Before any information you have gained is shared with other people the **service user's permission** must be obtained. If the reasons why you want to share the information is made clear to the service user, then consent is more likely to be given.

More detailed coverage of matters of confidentiality is given in Unit 1.

### Cultural differences

The language that service users speak in their own home and community is called their first language. To be able to communicate with people from different communities it is important to understand their cultural practices and religious beliefs.

It is important that services users have access to interpreters and advocates to act on their behalf when using care services. Interpreters will interpret what they are saying for you so you can understand and respond and advocates will help them gain access to services and act on their behalf to obtain their rights within the service. Advocates speak on behalf of service users and represent their interests. They listen and interpret for the service user. Language interpreters only translate the services users words into the language that the carer speaks.

## TASK

### How to apply the care values

Choose three components of the care value base and give examples of how you could apply them in practice in a care setting.

### Service users' rights and choices

It is very important that carers support the service users' rights and choices by implementing the care values and monitoring how they work out in practice so as to improve the service.

## Communicate effectively with service users

- Remember the care values when communicating with service users
- When working with service users always try to be thoughtful, considerate, kind, gentle and caring.

### Greeting service users

The way you address people is all-important. Ask them what they would like you to call them – Mr/Mrs or by their first name. Be aware of the service user's abilities, likes, dislikes, culture and religion.

Remember that, when welcoming services users to your particular care setting, they are likely to be feeling very nervous. Remember also that you are already familiar with the processes of the service and that you need to explain everything you do to the user to make them feel comfortable.

*Greeting a service user*

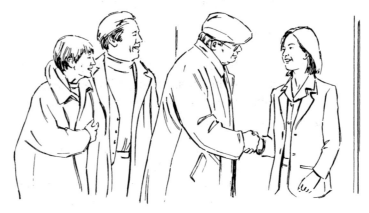

To make the experience as less frightening as possible for the service user:

- Remember that each service user is special, unique and with their own needs and expectations
- Welcome them warmly and make their relatives or friends welcome
- Tell the service user who you are, what you are going to do (for example make them a cup of tea and then take them to their room to settle in before you fill in an admission form)
- Remember what you have been told about body language – using positive body language will make them feel welcome and trust you
- Actively listen to what they have to say, and also their relatives or friends.

## Behaviours helpful to you when communicating in a group

- **Questioning** – Seeking information, opinion and ideas
- **Listening** – Showing verbally and non-verbally that you are paying attention and understand what others are saying
- **Informing** – Giving helpful information, opinions and ideas
- **Clarifying** – Clearing up confusion, defining terms and pointing out alternatives
- **Sharing** – Inviting comments using listening skills, keeping the communication channels open and making people feel involved
- **Supporting** – Recognising the individual rights, choices and identity of group members

*Formal group*

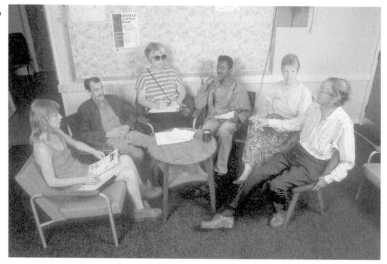

*Informal group*

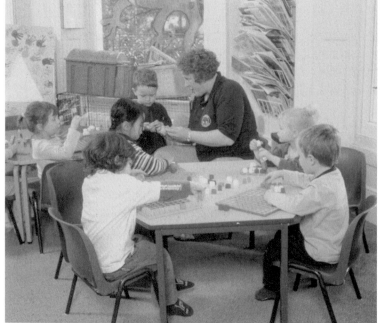

- **Encouraging** – Helping those who are shy, nervous or reluctant to contribute; this involves being friendly, warm and responsive, both verbally and non-verbally

- **Harmonising** – Recalling disagreements, reducing tension and getting people to explore their differences constructively

- **Asserting** – Using the rules of assertion, particularly in negotiation, to promote clarity and accuracy

- **Constructive disagreement** – Not upsetting people when there are disagreements. Other people's viewpoints may be incorporated into your own, so that the discussion becomes constructive. Focus first on what is agreed before disagreements are dealt with

- **Humour** – Reduces tension

- **Relaxation** – Creating an atmosphere of calmness and confidence

- **Cohesion** – Referring to the group as a team rather than as a collection of individuals.

## The support needed for effective communication in a group.

In order for interaction to be effective, the situation within which the interaction takes place must be as supportive as possible. This essentially means removing as many sources of stress from the situation as possible. This may be achieved by doing the following:

- Clearly introduce yourself

- Clearly introduce any others present

- Provide information about the background to the interaction

- Ensure that the physical environment is suitable, in that it is confidential and private, not noisy and uncomfortable

- The arrangement of seating should not reflect perceptions of power (e.g. one chair higher than another, or one participant behind a desk)

- All participants should have a clear view of each other

- Establish rapport, making full use of non-verbal behaviour

- Use open questions and self-disclosure where appropriate

- Use reflective listening

- Ensure that all the participants' uncertainties are resolved before concluding.

All the skills explained in this unit, whether in relation to individuals or groups, share the common objective of optimising the support of the interaction and reducing the anxieties of participants.

In addition, care values should always be applied. This means that the individuality of the participants is to be respected and responded to positively. Examples include arranging for translation where appropriate, respecting opinions that differ from your own and showing patience towards those who have communication difficulties.

## Evaluate the range of communication skills used and plan for improvements

### How can you evaluate your own communication skills?

It is important that you have some measure by which you can evaluate how effective your interpersonal interactions are. Listening is an important way of finding out how effective you are. We shall be examining in this section some techniques that you may wish to consider. Specific training in interpersonal skills is essential for work in care. This will provide the opportunity, in relatively safe situations, of experimenting and practising.

You can evaluate your own communication by monitoring:

- The quality of your contribution
- Improvement from previous occasions
- Your knowledge and understanding.

This monitoring should be done using a variety of methods:

- Verbal feedback may be obtained from the individual with whom you are interacting, or an observer, or both.
- Written feedback is best obtained from an independent observer, who may rate you against specific criteria (e.g. how many open questions were used).
- Video observation is useful, because you can observe your own behaviour and may observe things that you missed when in the process of interacting. An advantage of video observation is that you can watch it again and again.
- Self-reflection is useful in addition to the above three observational techniques. It is worth recording your own experience of the interview in some detail.

The process of writing it down often makes things clearer. A traditional training method in social care work is called 'process recording', which is a very detailed self-reflection on service user interviews.

Observation of interaction is vital to understanding. Not just observing and reflecting on your own skills but observing others is also extremely valuable, and using video will allow you to evaluate your own interpersonal effectiveness and that of other care workers. Taking a step back to evaluate develops care workers' sensitivity to the interpersonal world around them. Ultimately, the care worker assumes a primary professional responsibility for the success of the interaction.

*Checklist to evaluate your own communication skills.*

| Skill | How well did you do? – Write notes on your performance |
|---|---|
| Clearness of speech | |
| Pace of speech | |
| Tone of voice | |
| Asking open questions | |
| Asking closed questions | |
| Clarifying | |
| Respecting silence | |
| Empathy | |
| Assertive behaviour | |
| Using prompts | |
| Reflection of content of situation | |
| Paraphrasing | |
| Summarising | |

The care worker must address any misunderstanding on the part of the service user.

Effective interaction requires reflective practice, and even the most advanced practitioners are continually striving to improve their skills.

## Evaluate your interpersonal communication skills

For this task, you must collect information on how effective your own skills are in a one-to-one interaction. By doing this, you will begin to develop the skills of reflective practice.

1. Select a service user with whom you can have a useful interaction. The interaction can be a formal interview, although a more informal interaction would be just as acceptable. Interact with the service user for a period of time (a minimum of 10 minutes is suggested).
2. Make notes during the interaction. These notes will be about the interaction, not about the service user. If making notes during the interview is uncomfortable, ask someone to do it for you, or use a video camera to record the interview so that you can make notes afterwards.

Organise your observations under five headings:

1. **Factors in the environment** – Describe the immediate environment within which the interaction occurred. You will want to describe the room, the seating arrangement, the time of day and whether anyone else was present.
2. **Body language** – Describe your body language. For example, you should discuss your posture, gestures, facial expressions, body contact, personal space and eye contact.
3. **Interpersonal skills** – Describe in as much detail as possible what skills you have used (for example open questions), and provide specific examples for each skill identified. Your examples could include your spoken words, as well as a description of your tone of voice. Try not to just give examples, but explain why specific skills were chosen. Identify as many skills as you can.
4. **Enhancing factors** – Describe the physical, emotional and social factors that helped to make the interaction effective – Refer to the relevant sections of this unit for examples of what sorts of factor you can describe. Be sure to explain why any factor you have identified as enhancing made the interaction more effective.
5. **Inhibiting factors** – Describe the physical, emotional and social factors that made the interaction less effective than it might have been, and why.

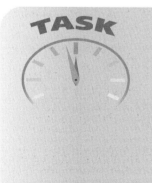

## Plan to improve your interpersonal communication skills

You have already evaluated your communication skills and made suggestions about how they might be improved. Now you must develop an action plan that you can use to help develop your communication skills. In order to develop the action plan, you need to do several things.

1. For each of the communication skills you have identified as needing improvement, clearly state what best practice would consist of. It is best practice that you will be aiming for.

2. Your action plan should then clearly explain how you might develop your communication skills from where they are currently to best practice. You will want to explain how opportunities for supervised practice, as well as training, can be used to develop your skills. You may also want to consider the use of keeping reflective journals, as well as reading books on interpersonal skills. You may want to consider more advanced approaches such as NLP, or learning counselling skills.

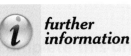

**further information**

Adams R (1994) *Skilled Work with People*. Collins Educational, London

Clarke L (2000) *Health and Social Care for Foundation GNVQ*. Nelson Thornes, Cheltenham

Clarke L (2000) *Health and Social Care for Intermediate GNVQ*. Nelson Thornes, Cheltenham

Clarke L (2002) *Health and Social Care GCSE*. Nelson Thornes, Cheltenham

Clarke L, White M and Rowell K (2002) *An Entry Level Course in Caring*. Nelson Thornes, Cheltenham

Green S (2002) *BTEC National Early Years*. Nelson Thornes, Cheltenham

Nolan Y (2003) *Care. NVQ Level 2 Student Handbook*, 2nd edn. Heinemann, Oxford

Pease A (1989) *Body Language*. Sheldon Press, London

## Summary

- Oral communication can be encouraged by carers' physical responses to service users. Eye contact, smiling, sympathetic listening and responses will all help.

- Some of the skills needed for effective communication are active listening, appropriate responses, knowing when to keep quiet, knowing how to ask questions and appropriate non-verbal behaviour.

- Effective listening is a vital part of effective communication. Carers should try and reflect on what the person has said and how they said it and should not feel awkward if there are a lot of silences.

- Carers should not allow personal values and attitudes to dictate how they communicate with service users.

- Initial contact and ways of greeting service users and their families are

- That your personal problems are affecting your work and attitude towards service users
- Tired and impatient
- Immature and unable to understand a service user's problem
- That you have difficulty in forming relationships with service users or colleagues
- Worried because the demands of your job are excessive overwhelmed with paperwork
- Not trained enough for the demands of the job.

Perhaps you can think of other issues that might arise?

Sometimes you may feel overwhelmed by the responsibilities and tasks you are expected to carry out. It is at times like this, when you are under stress, that it is most important that you remember and work with the care values in mind. Care values are principles, standards or qualities considered worthwhile or desirable by the care profession.

## The social care values

Social care values address three elements:

- Fostering individuality and diversity
- Maintaining confidentiality
- Fostering rights and beliefs.

*Empowering service users*

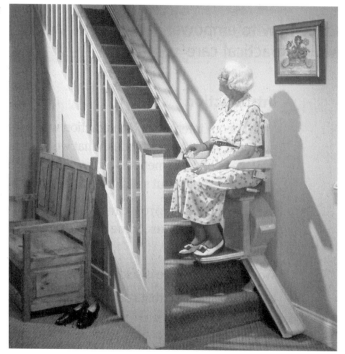

The intention of having care values is to create equality, dignity and respect for all individuals. Use of these care values help to empower service users. Care workers should:

- Identify and question his/her own values and prejudices, and their implications for practice
- Respect and value uniqueness and diversity, and recognise and build on strengths
- Promote people's rights to choice, privacy, confidentiality and protection while recognising and addressing the complexities of competing rights and demands
- Assist people to increase control of, and improve the quality of, their lives while recognising that control of behaviour will be required at times in order to protect people from harm
- Identify, analyse and take action to counter discrimination, racism, disadvantage, inequality and injustice, using strategies appropriate to the situation
- Practise in a manner that does not stigmatise or disadvantage individuals, groups or communities.

## How do you apply the care values?

### Foster individual rights and beliefs

Unless you treat each person as an individual you are likely to make assumptions about them – that is, you may make a judgement about them based on something you have seen or read. The judgement may be wrong but it affects your interaction with that person. The assumption grows to a stereotype – we make the person fit the image we have of them rather than accepting them for what they are.

In Unit 2 we looked at how stereotypes can inhibit effective communication and act as barriers to good communication. Good carers try to be aware of the stereotypes that they believe in, particularly when the person they are trying to help is from a different social class, from a different ethnic background or of the opposite gender.

Here are some examples of how we can easily misjudge people and get the wrong message.

- **Judging on appearance** – 'The guy looked so punk I thought he was very threatening but he was really gentle when he worked with the toddlers.' Day nursery assistant
- **Judging age** – 'Old people don't care about their appearance so I don't bother if the hem of Doris's underskirt falls below her dress or Pop walks around with his fly undone.' Care assistant in elderly persons' home
- **Judging disabled people (see the wheelchair and assume total immobility)** – 'I was really surprised when I pushed the wheelchair to

the toilet block and she got up and walked to the toilet on her own.' College tutor who has just had a disabled student join a course

- **Judging academic ability to be the same as emotional and social ability** – 'Some of them are so slow you wouldn't think they'd be interested in anything romantic.' Student working alongside some other students with learning difficulties.

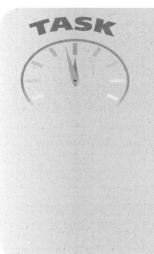

**Case Study**

An old people's home offering respite care or temporary care for elderly people while relatives have a break admitted a woman from a Moslem background. The staff could have assumed that she wouldn't mind just eating like everyone else for her short stay. They could have assumed that she was no longer practising her religion. They did, however, check her dietary requirements and took trouble to obtain the right food. This made a huge difference to her stay.

*Examine your own prejudices – being aware of them is halfway to overcoming them.*

**TASK**

### Empowering service users when providing practical care

Give examples of four ways that service users can be empowered. Describe how care workers can apply the care values when working with service users. You must provide an example of implementation of all three components of the care values (fostering individuality and diversity, confidentiality and fostering rights and beliefs).

When carrying out these tasks it is important that you consider that your own attitudes and opinions might influence any actions that take place with service users. It is also important that you give an example of how service users make their own decisions and how you provide information to allow then to make such decisions.

**AO2** ## Review the skills and qualities that contribute to effective practical caring

There are many skills that a carer can use when supporting in a practical way the needs of service users. You need to be patient and to have understanding and respect for service users' needs. You also need to have the qualities of a sense of humour, cheerfulness and a willingness to do things for the service user.

## Interpersonal skills

How you use interpersonal skill to support service users is discussed in more detail in Unit 2.

## Patience

Carers need patience when supporting service users – people who cannot speak or who have other disabilities may not be very quick in carrying out tasks such as dressing themselves, getting in or out of bed or getting into or out of a wheelchair.

Many service users have difficulty with self-care, such as cutting toenails, bathing, showering or washing all over, feeding, brushing hair or shaving.

How can you maintain the service user's independence and dignity?

One of the ways in which we can support service users to maintain their dignity and independence is to give them choice and allow them to make decisions that affect their lives.

*Be sensitive to service users' needs*

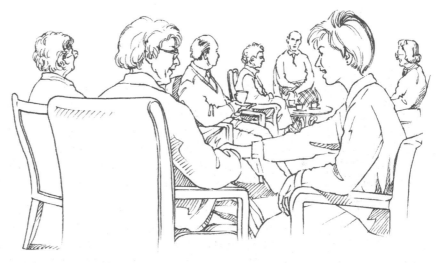

Giving this choice is central to the quality of care. It takes the power and control from the carer and places it where it belongs, with the service user. Society – that is, we – tends not to listen to people who have disabilities. However, by offering choice to people we empower them. This gives them a sense of dignity and worth.

We can empower service users by:

- Being sensitive to their needs
- Listening to what they are saying
- Not 'talking down' to them
- Not labelling those people with disabilities
- Negotiating with the service user, carer and any other professionals
- Giving appropriate support as necessary.

## Interpersonal communication

The development of your interpersonal skills is discussed in detail in Unit 2.

While working with service users it is useful to take the opportunity to observe how other workers interact with people and learn from them. Really, there is hardly a minute that cannot be used to gain some knowledge.

Use your observation skills also to help you to respond effectively to people:

- Is the person happy, sad, and dejected?
- What is the person's attitude to other people and to his or her surroundings?
- Is the person anxious or tense?
- Can the person see?
- Can the person hear?
- Can the person talk or is signing used?

## Listening

Listen actively. Get ready to listen. Make the shift from speaker to listener a complete one. You must really focus and try to remember what the person has said. A good listener hears the content of what the speaker says and the intent – what the person means.

## How we can use empathy to help people

As you listen actively and try to reflect back to the person their feelings and what they say, you will gradually move towards empathy. That is, you

*Empathy can establish trust between carer and service user*

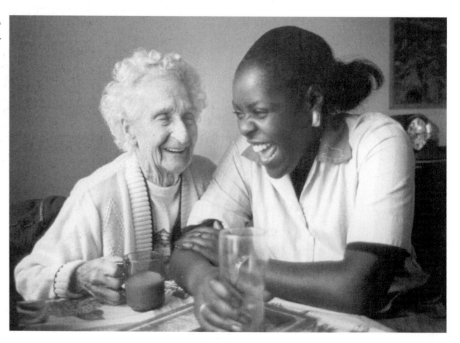

will be able to put yourself in the other person's position. You need to empathise in order to be able to help the person effectively.

One important aspect of providing support to any service user is to do so in a way that maintains the service user's independence and dignity.

To help people in a sensitive and caring manner, remember that you will need to pay constant attention to the way you talk to them. Be polite and respectful when talking to them and talk in a clear voice. Always talk to the person about what you are doing and why. This will help them to feel at ease and understand what you are doing.

Aim to:

- Listen and respond to communications from service users
- Use good eye contact and keep smiling
- Be sincere, sympathetic and understanding
- Be kind, gentle and tactful
- Be willing to assist, but always allow the person to do as much as possible for themselves
- Encourage them to be as independent as practical.

*Ensure that service users are as independent as possible*

When working with people with disabilities it is important to be careful not to oppress them. You could do this by exercising power over their lives, by doing things for them or by making decisions for them. The language used to describe dependent people can be oppressive. For example, labelling everyone over the age of 65 as 'elderly' can be damaging to their self-esteem or self-confidence.

### Scientific

Carers will be called upon to perform a number of scientific tasks depending on their role.

Residential carers may be called upon to clean, disinfect and sterilise equipment such as instruments, trays, bedpans, etc.

### Practical

Carers not only need good interpersonal and communication skills, they also need the ability to apply themselves to practical tasks.

Tasks such as cleaning, disinfecting and sterilising equipment are important skills that are a requisite of a good carer.

It is also important that the carers can perform practical tasks such as cleaning, making beds, washing service users and supporting them with daily living activities.

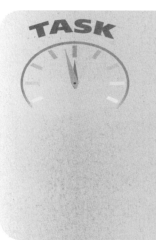

**TASK**

## Reviewing the skills and qualities that contribute to effective practical caring

To allow service users to make their own decisions carers will need to exercise their skill to empower the service users.

To show that you can use these skills effectively you must chose three or four practical tasks and give examples of how you would use skills such as patience, understanding, empathy, respect, sense of humour and cheerfulness to support service users.

You should also discuss how these qualities would help to build up good relationships with service users.

 **AO3**

## Provide support for service users when choosing clothing, dressing and putting on outer garments

### Choice

It is important that service users should have a choice as to what they wear and when they wear it. It would not empower service users if they were told what to wear or had little choice. It is therefore very important that you should discuss the kinds of clothes, style and fabrics that service users like to wear.

Some service users may need advice about the different types of clothes available to them; for example, a person who is incontinent will need information about the different incontinence products and types of clothing available so as to be able to make an informed choice.

Other service users may be allergic to certain kinds of fabric, which may cause rashes or other reactions.

The range of equipment available to dependent people, either in their own homes or in residential care, is vast.

## Why do people need help with practical daily living activities?

The quality of life of a service user will depend to some extent on their being able to move around freely without pain, discomfort or danger. We all take mobility (a person's ability to walk, wash, dress, feed themselves, etc.) for granted from the time we first learn to walk.

If a person's mobility is reduced, the scope of their daily life can become severely limited, as they may be unable to get out of bed, wash or feed themselves. A number of service users will need physical assistance with daily living activities, such as eating, walking, hearing or seeing. This support and assistance has to be provided safely and using equipment such as wheelchairs, walking frames and hearing aids where necessary.

Many factors contribute to loss of, or reduced, mobility in elderly people:

- Arthritis
- Strokes
- Breathing problems
- Heart conditions
- Foot problems.

Many of these problems can be alleviated by assertive aids to mobility. Assertive equipment includes wheelchairs, walking frames, hoists, specially designed knives, spoons, forks, etc.

Assertive equipment falls into the following categories:

- Personal care support
- Hoists and lifting equipment
- Eating and drinking aids
- Help with dressing and undressing
- Mobility aids
- Reading and hearing aids.

How can the use of assertive equipment when dressing help a dependent person to live as independent a life as possible? Assertive equipment improves the service user's ability to carry out certain tasks such as dressing themselves with dignity without a carer being present. It is important that service users wear their own clothes when in residential care and not clothes supplied without consultation and choice by the establishment. Carers should do all possible to meet the wishes of the service user. People express their individuality through the clothes they

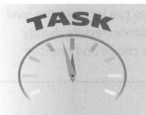

## Assistive devices for personal care

There are regional disability centres where a range of assistive devices for personal care is on display, e.g. Disability North in Newcastle. Where is your nearest regional disability centre?

Make arrangements to visit your regional centre. These organisations allow visitors to see aids and also to try them out. While you are there, see if you can collect any leaflets and catalogues which will help you to illustrate your portfolio work and deepen your understanding of the range of aids available.

Visit a local care setting near you. Ask to see the types of assistive aids they have.

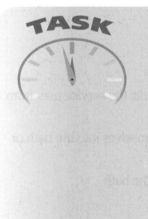

## Support for service users when choosing clothing and when dressing

Give two examples of how you would use your skills to encourage service users to take part in choosing their own clothing to maintain their appearance.

Explain how shoehorns, stocking aids, sock aids and Velcro could be used to support service users when they are dressing.

You will be observed supporting one service user in choosing and putting on an item of outer clothing. You must perform this task independently, confidently and competently.

You should also keep a logbook that shows the theoretical reasons for the actions you have taken.

 **AO4** **Investigate and provide support for service users to maintain and improve mobility**

### The benefits of remaining mobile

Before a mobility aid is offered to a service user they will usually have been seen by an occupational therapist or physiotherapist to assess their need for such an appliance. This professional will discuss the situation with the service user and watch them carrying out their usual activities so as to be able to recommend the most appropriate aid. Service users also need support in the correct way to use the aid. To misuse an aid could cause injury.

Mobility aids or appliances help the service user to continue to be mobile. Aids such as walking sticks and walking frames help those service users

Other service users may be allergic to certain kinds of fabric, which may cause rashes or other reactions.

The range of equipment available to dependent people, either in their own homes or in residential care, is vast.

## Why do people need help with practical daily living activities?

The quality of life of a service user will depend to some extent on their being able to move around freely without pain, discomfort or danger. We all take mobility (a person's ability to walk, wash, dress, feed themselves, etc.) for granted from the time we first learn to walk.

If a person's mobility is reduced, the scope of their daily life can become severely limited, as they may be unable to get out of bed, wash or feed themselves. A number of service users will need physical assistance with daily living activities, such as eating, walking, hearing or seeing. This support and assistance has to be provided safely and using equipment such as wheelchairs, walking frames and hearing aids where necessary.

Many factors contribute to loss of, or reduced, mobility in elderly people:

- Arthritis
- Strokes
- Breathing problems
- Heart conditions
- Foot problems.

Many of these problems can be alleviated by assertive aids to mobility. Assertive equipment includes wheelchairs, walking frames, hoists, specially designed knives, spoons, forks, etc.

Assertive equipment falls into the following categories:

- Personal care support
- Hoists and lifting equipment
- Eating and drinking aids
- Help with dressing and undressing
- Mobility aids
- Reading and hearing aids.

How can the use of assertive equipment when dressing help a dependent person to live as independent a life as possible? Assertive equipment improves the service user's ability to carry out certain tasks such as dressing themselves with dignity without a carer being present. It is important that service users wear their own clothes when in residential care and not clothes supplied without consultation and choice by the establishment. Carers should do all possible to meet the wishes of the service user. People express their individuality through the clothes they wear and feel empowered when they can make their own choices about the way they present themselves.

*Examples of dressing aids*

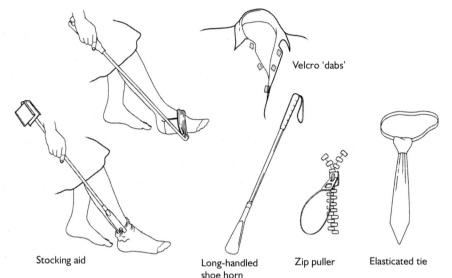

Stocking aid

Velcro 'dabs'

Long-handled shoe horn

Zip puller

Elasticated tie

## Help with dressing

Service users sometimes have problems with dressing and undressing. These are simple tasks, but can be made difficult by even the slightest disability, such as a broken finger or a muscle strain. Arthritic joints make it difficult to do up buttons or lift the arms above the head. Service users can use Velcro instead of zips or buttons, and a number of other aids to dressing can be used, as shown in the illustration above.

### Hair care

Aids that can assist in hair care include:

● Hair brushes and combs with extra long handles

● Wheelchair shampoo tray – the shape fits around the service user's neck, allowing water to drain into the sink without getting the service user wet

● Inflatable hair wash brush – designed for washing the hair of someone confined to bed.

### Foot care

Assistive devices include long-reach nail scissors, to prevent excessive bending.

Remember:

● Make sure that people can dress in privacy

- Make sure that service users have enough information to make a choice about their clothing
- Do not choose a service user's clothes – always involve them in making the decisions.

The quality of life for a service user will depend to some extent on being able to move around freely, without pain, discomfort or danger. Most of us take mobility for granted. If a person's mobility is reduced, the scope of that person's daily life can become severely limited as the ability to complete personal care becomes impaired.

A number of service users will need physical assistance with daily living activities such as changing clothes.

Care users may need assistance in personal care for a variety of reasons:

- Learning disability
- A physical disability which restricts movement.

Many factors contribute to loss of, or reduced, mobility in elderly people:

- Arthritis
- Strokes
- Breathing problems
- Heart conditions/disorders
- Foot problems – e.g. as a result of diabetes.

Other care users may need practical support in personal care because of:

- Illness
- Dementia.

## Types of assistance

The types of assistance service users may need with personal hygiene can vary. Care workers need to respect the dignity of the service user at all times. It is a good idea to encourage the service user's independence or, if this is not possible, them to take part in the washing routine. Ask the service user for permission before helping with washing and bathing and try to establish a regular personal hygiene routine. Some service users may not want a bath every day while others may prefer a shower. Where someone is confined to bed, a bed bath can help them stay clean, fresh and comfortable. Always explain what you are doing and cover any parts of the body you are not cleaning to protect the service user from embarrassment. Screens, if available, should be drawn around the bed and doors need to be closed when cleaning procedures are taking place.

Hair care involves regular shampooing, conditioning, styling and cutting. Some care settings encourage the use of hairdressers, as good self-image can be very helpful to a sense of well-being. Male service users may need support with shaving. It is also important to make sure that hair is free from head lice or nits. Foot care involves washing feet, cutting toenails, checking against fungicidal infections and treating corns and bunions. Massaging feet is very important as blood flow to the feet may be restricted as a result of some medical conditions such as diabetes or heart disease. It is important to test the temperature of the water, as scalding is very common – sometimes service users cannot gauge the water temperature correctly as they may have little feeling in their feet.

Good oral hygiene is also important. This can involve brushing teeth or cleaning dentures. Any thick coating on the tongue or blisters on gums should be recorded and appropriate treatment sought. Dentists and chiropodists visit care centres to help older people with teeth and feet problems.

Service users may also need help when changing clothing. Some service users have arthritis and find it very difficult to bend down, for example to put socks on. Some dementia sufferers may need help to work out which clothes to put on and in what order. Clothes are very often labelled in care settings and service users need to retain the choice of which clothes to wear.

Any assistance with personal hygiene can provide the care worker with an opportunity to chat to the service user and build up a relationship of trust, friendliness and caring.

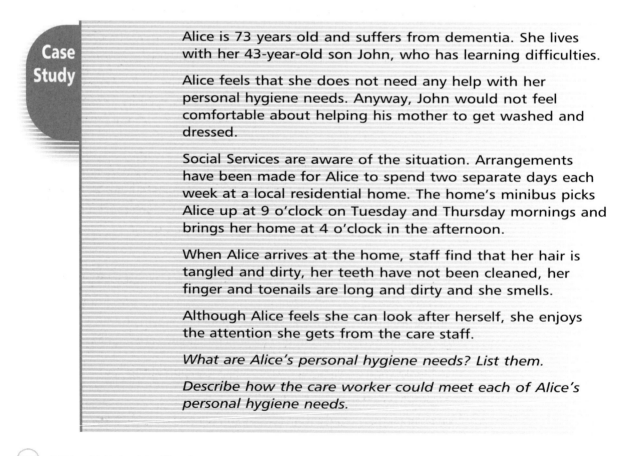

**Case Study**

Alice is 73 years old and suffers from dementia. She lives with her 43-year-old son John, who has learning difficulties.

Alice feels that she does not need any help with her personal hygiene needs. Anyway, John would not feel comfortable about helping his mother to get washed and dressed.

Social Services are aware of the situation. Arrangements have been made for Alice to spend two separate days each week at a local residential home. The home's minibus picks Alice up at 9 o'clock on Tuesday and Thursday mornings and brings her home at 4 o'clock in the afternoon.

When Alice arrives at the home, staff find that her hair is tangled and dirty, her teeth have not been cleaned, her finger and toenails are long and dirty and she smells.

Although Alice feels she can look after herself, she enjoys the attention she gets from the care staff.

*What are Alice's personal hygiene needs? List them.*

*Describe how the care worker could meet each of Alice's personal hygiene needs.*

## Application of the care values in care

Care values are principles, standards or qualities considered worthwhile or desirable by the care profession. If you work in the health and social care field it is important to pay them a great deal of attention. Care values to think about include the following:

- **Fostering rights and diversity**

  - Service users' choice, preferences and wishes must be respected

  - People must not be judged because of their culture, race, religion, sexual identity, age, gender, health status, etc.

- **Maintaining confidentiality**

  - Service users have the right to say who should have access to personal data

  - Care workers are responsible for respecting the wishes of the service user.

- **Fostering rights and beliefs**

  - Service users' choice, preferences and wishes must be respected

  - Each individual's own personal beliefs and preferences – religious, cultural, political, ethical and sexual – must be respected

  - Listen to other individuals

  - Promote effective communication in a variety of ways

  - Consider language (verbal and non-verbal), understanding, environment, and social and cultural influences.

All these issues are known together as the care values. It is hoped that by stimulating thought and discussion through training and exposing carers to a wide variety of situations, attitudes may be developed that are consistent with this value base.

Care values involve respect for:

- Individual rights, for example the service user should be able to refuse to accept the help we offer

- Personal beliefs such as religion – food, dress, etc.

- Race

- Confidentiality – not to divulge anything the service user tells you without their permission

- The way we communicate with people.

People who work in social care should:

- Identify and question their own values and prejudices

- Respect and value individuality in people

- Promote people's rights to choice, privacy and confidentiality

- Assist people to gain control of, and improve the quality of, their lives
- Identify and take action to deal with discrimination, racism, disadvantage, inequality and injustice
- Carry out their job in a way that does not disadvantage either individuals, groups or communities.

Here are some examples of the care values in practice.

Table 3.1

| Care value | Application to personal care needs |
|---|---|
| Anti-discriminatory practice | Some service users may be considered 'high risk' e.g. HIV service users. Care must be taken to treat all people with the same respect and care<br>A care user may have a hearing disability.<br>The care worker must treat all service users sensitively |
| Confidentiality | Care workers have access to confidential information about service users. They must not abuse this position of trust by gossiping to others about service users |
| Promoting choice | The service user is given the choice (where possible) of whether to have a bath or not and when to have one<br>The service user is given the choice about what clothes to wear<br>Assistance with daily living activities and the use of assistive equipment helps to increase the service user's level of independence and provides more opportunities for choice<br>'New build' care homes for older people often have 'en suite' bathing facilities. This also increases the level of choice |
| Promoting personal beliefs and identity | Care workers need to know different customs and belief systems. Some cultures do not allow total immersion in water (bathing); other cultures do not wash hair often or cut hair<br>Some religions do not allow female service users to be washed by male care workers<br>Care workers must respect the belief systems of others |
| Effective communication | Care workers can talk to their service users about their personal hygiene needs and offer support and care in an understanding and sincere way |

▶

| Practical support | The use of assistive devices can increase the level of service users' independence, restore dignity and self-esteem, promote choice and improve quality of life |
| --- | --- |

## Aids that allow service users greater independence in their personal hygiene

Assistive devices are aids to everyday living that can help people to be more independent and improve their quality of life. The range of equipment available to people in care settings is vast. It varies from small, inexpensive items such as special long-handled toenail clippers to very large, expensive pieces of equipment such as hoists, wheelchairs and stair lifts.

### Bathing

Aids to assist bathing include:

- Hand rails and grips in bathrooms and showers
- An extra-grip rubber mat in the bath that prevents the service user from slipping
- A bath seat that allows the person to swing themselves into the bath or shower
- A bath hoist – to lift the person into and out of the bath
- A powered bath lift.

Other aids that are available to make bathing easier, especially where there is some restricted limb movement, include inflatable bath pillows for comfort, a step stool to make it easier to get into the bath and a long-handled sponge.

Service users and care workers can be injured if equipment, even the right equipment, is not properly maintained. Service providers must make sure that all equipment is in good working order and is regularly checked for safety, and that staff are trained in its correct use.

*Aids to assist bathing*

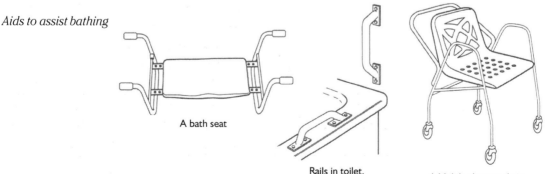

A bath seat

Rails in toilet, bath and shower

A Mobile shower chair

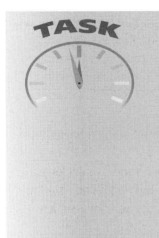

## Assistive devices for personal care

There are regional disability centres where a range of assistive devices for personal care is on display, e.g. Disability North in Newcastle. Where is your nearest regional disability centre?

Make arrangements to visit your regional centre. These organisations allow visitors to see aids and also to try them out. While you are there, see if you can collect any leaflets and catalogues which will help you to illustrate your portfolio work and deepen your understanding of the range of aids available.

Visit a local care setting near you. Ask to see the types of assistive aids they have.

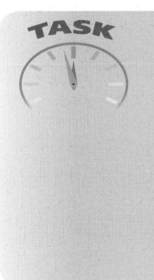

## Support for service users when choosing clothing and when dressing

Give two examples of how you would use your skills to encourage service users to take part in choosing their own clothing to maintain their appearance.

Explain how shoehorns, stocking aids, sock aids and Velcro could be used to support service users when they are dressing.

You will be observed supporting one service user in choosing and putting on an item of outer clothing. You must perform this task independently, confidently and competently.

You should also keep a logbook that shows the theoretical reasons for the actions you have taken.

 **AO4** **Investigate and provide support for service users to maintain and improve mobility**

### The benefits of remaining mobile

Before a mobility aid is offered to a service user they will usually have been seen by an occupational therapist or physiotherapist to assess their need for such an appliance. This professional will discuss the situation with the service user and watch them carrying out their usual activities so as to be able to recommend the most appropriate aid. Service users also need support in the correct way to use the aid. To misuse an aid could cause injury.

Mobility aids or appliances help the service user to continue to be mobile. Aids such as walking sticks and walking frames help those service users who may be frail or unsteady on their feet to move about. Use of these aids can also help a service user become more confident or help them to regain confidence.

Always check on the condition of a mobility aid before you give it to a service users and afterwards on a regular basis.

## Walking sticks

For people who need extra support when walking, a variety of sticks are available. They are usually made from aluminium and can be adjusted in length or folded. Variations include tripod and quadruped sticks, which provide extra stability, and traditional, wooden sticks which are still popular. Seat sticks are useful, being made of lightweight aluminium and can be turned into a seat when the user wants to rest for short periods.

Walking sticks need to be measured to fit the service user. There are a number of different kinds of walking stick. An adjustable walking stick, usually metal, can be adjusted by sliding the inner section up or down until the correct height is found for the person using the stick. Wooden walking sticks need to be cut to the correct length and a rubber ferrule placed at the end so that it does not slip.

*A selection of crutches and walking frames*

## Tripod

Service users who have difficulty in walking on one particular leg should only use a tripod.

When using the tripod it should be positioned in the hand opposite to the leg that needs support. If the left leg is the one that needs support then the tripod should be held in the right hand.

## Zimmer or walking frame

Zimmers are the best-known type of walking frame. Frames give good support, enabling service users to stand or walk on their own. There are also adjustable walkers or frames, which have two fixed wheels at the front and two rubber feet at the back. They can be adjusted in height so that the user can rest their arms on the frame.

## Crutches

For people who are unable to bear their own weight or who need extra support when walking, a range of lightweight, aluminium elbow crutches are available. The height can be adjusted to suit the individual. It is important that service users and carers should understand the correct way to use crutches and a physiotherapist will usually advise on this.

## Wheelchairs

These may be electronically-controlled, hand-propelled by the service user or pushed by a helper. Various accessories are available including trays, soft seats, safety straps and spring lifter seats. The amount of help a wheelchair user will need obviously depends on the type of service user involved. Remember that the aim is to encourage mobility as far as possible. Never take over if a service user wants to try to move unaided.

*Examples of hand-propelled and powered wheelchairs*

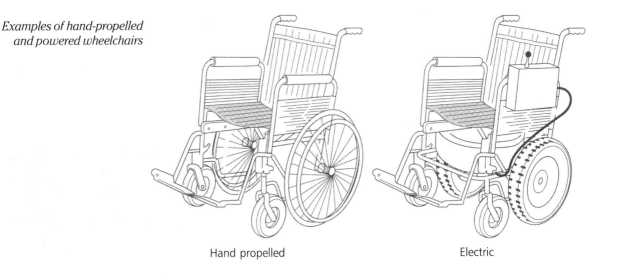

Hand propelled                                        Electric

### Correct use of wheelchairs

Service users should only use wheelchairs that have been correctly measured and assessed by a carer such as an occupational therapist or physiotherapist. Young service users may have their own views about the type of wheelchair they prefer, the colour it should be and additions it should have.

The steps that should be used when assisting service users in wheelchairs are as follows.

1. Assess the situation and decide what is going to be required.

2. Explain to the service user what is going to happen.

3. Look at the chair carefully to establish the position of the brake, the foot rests, the armrests and any safety straps.

4. Always ensure that the user is comfortably and, more importantly, safely seated.

5. Make sure that arms and legs are positioned carefully in order to avoid knocks on doorways and other obstacles.

6. When negotiating steps and kerbs, place your foot on the tipping lever, hold the chair firmly and tip it back to go up.

7. Lower the chair down the kerb; the back wheels should touch the ground at the same time.

8. If you are pushing a wheelchair, never go too quickly as this can be frightening for the service user.

9 When transferring service users to and from wheelchairs, make sure the brakes are firmly applied, footrests are turned out of the way, small front wheels are turned inwards and the appropriate arm of the chair is removed.

Remember that some users may wish to use a cushion to minimise the risk of pressure sores.

Do not assume that people who use wheelchairs need help and support to get about.

## Hoists and lifting equipment

Hoists and lifting equipment not only help maintain the independence of the service user, but they are also an enormous help to the carers. They make lifting safer and easier. Some hoists are fixed, perhaps beside a person's bed or bath, but most are portable. This means that they can be used in a number of situations in the home with safety. They may be either manually or electrically operated.

*Bath hoist and stair lift*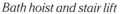

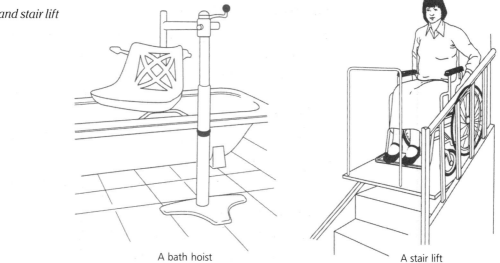

A bath hoist                                A stair lift

## Other mobility aids

Handrails allow the service user to walk unaided in bathrooms or toilets. The rail also allows elderly people to lower themselves on to the toilet. Sometimes a raised toilet seat also helps.

A bath seat allows the person to swing themselves, on their own, into a bath or shower, thus helping to preserve their dignity and self-respect.

## What are the main sources of assistive equipment?

There are four main sources from which service users or their families or carers can obtain aids to daily living and adaptations to make it safer and easier in their own homes.

### Where can a service user get information?

There are centres where people can go to see aids and adaptations and try them out. These centres are provided by:

- Some Social Services departments
- Some of the larger chemist chains
- Voluntary organisations, such as the Spastics Society, the Red Cross or Help the Aged.

The DSS also provides a leaflet (reference no. HB 2) that gives information about centres and where people can get help.

On a national level, the Disabled Living Foundation (380–384 Harrow Road, London W9 2HU) runs a free information service for service users, their families or carers. They will either give helpful information or refer you to someone who can advise. They also have a permanent exhibition of aids and other equipment that can be tried out.

### Social Services departments

Since 1948 local authorities have had a responsibility to provide aids to daily living for people living in their own homes.

The increasing demand for support for those with a disability living in the community led to the Chronically Sick and Disabled Persons Act 1971. This stated that local authorities had a duty to find out the number of disabled people living in their area and their needs. The Act also stated that public buildings must have access for disabled people. Televisions and telephones might also be provided by Social Services departments.

Social Services departments now also have the responsibility for providing non-medical aids and equipment to help with everyday life. Aids are usually provided free, but in more and more cases there may be a charge. Wheelchairs may be loaned, as well as the more personal non-medical aids such as cutlery, eating aids, hoists, commodes and walking aids.

If you ask the local Social Services department for help, they will usually ask someone, such as an occupational therapist, to visit and discuss the suitability of the various aids available.

The Social Services departments can also alter a service user's home or put in some specialist equipment to help make life easier for them.

They can:

- Install hand rails in bathrooms, hallways and stairs
- Provide stair lifts
- Provide ramps for wheelchair access
- Widen doors
- Build specially designed bathrooms or toilets.

Service users usually make a financial contribution towards the costs of alterations or large adaptations.

### The National Health Service

Through the NHS the district nursing service can provide aids to help with home nursing, such as commodes, incontinence pads and bed aids. GPs can prescribe a number of medical aids, such as wheelchairs. Hospitals can also provide aids, such as support collars, callipers, wheelchairs, walking aids, hearing aids and low vision aids.

### Voluntary and private organisations

If some service users experience difficulty in getting appropriate aids, they can either be obtained from a voluntary organisation or bought from large chemists. Some voluntary organisations, such as the Red Cross, provide equipment and aids on short-term or long-term loan. They can supply such items as wheelchairs, commodes, bed rests, feeding cups, etc.

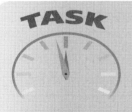

## TASK

## Support for service users to maintain and improve their mobility

Give three examples of how you would use your skills to encourage service users to use appropriate mobility aids and make informed judgements about the benefits to the service user of remaining mobile.

Explain how walking aids, Zimmer frame and tripod could be used to support service users to be mobile.

You will be observed demonstrating how to use mobility aids including a wheelchair in the correct way. You must perform these tasks independently, confidently and competently.

You should also keep a log book, which shows the theoretical reason for the actions you have taken.

**AO5** # Assist service users to choose meals and serve simple meals to service users

### Assisting service users to choose – the importance of a healthy diet

The important aspect of your diet is balancing what your body needs for it to work as you want it to, with what you eat and drink. In doing this you supply all that is needed for the body to function without building up too much stored fat or causing any deficiency disorder.

It would be easy to provide a balanced healthy diet if all the food you ate was made up of specific amounts of the required nutrients. This is the basis of many of the foods used by astronauts. However, no one food that you eat contains all the nutrients in the correct proportions.

If you are going to eat a balanced diet, you need to know:

● What your body needs – this depends upon your age, sex and activity level

● What nutrients are contained in the foods you eat.

However, most important of all is that everyone, professional workers and carers, must take into account, and act upon, the wishes of the service user. What the service user wants is the most important thing, not what is available to offer them or what we as carers might think is the best thing for them. It is the service user who must have the final say in what services and support they want.

So that the service user can make informed decisions about meals, the carer should:

● Explain what process they are involved in

● Let the service user put forward their own views

● Agree with the service user what services they would wish

● Talk through with the service user how the services can be delivered

● Involve the service user fully in reviewing the situation as appropriate.

### Why might people need support with eating and drinking?

They may have a physical disability, which could be short-term, such as a broken arm or wrist, or long-term, such as chronic arthritis. Because of their situation they may be unable to use a knife or fork or cup or cut their food.

They might have a sight disability and be unable to see their food.

Some people may lose their appetite because they are on medication, others because they are depressed. Some people may not like the food they are given.

To help people feed themselves, there are a number of aids available: cutlery, plates, trays, drinking aids. For example, service users with arthritis of the hand, which may cause poor grip, can have knives and forks with thick handles. Plates with rubber bases to stop the plate from slipping are useful for people with the use of only one hand.

*Aids to assisting eating and drinking*

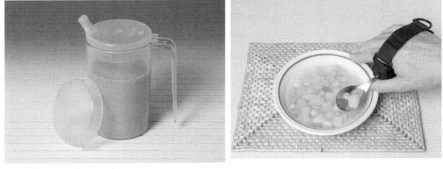

If, when you are helping a person to eat their food, something goes wrong you need to evaluate the situation and make a decision to deal with the situation yourself or request appropriate assistance.

- If a person is showing signs of choking, take the appropriate action (see pages 363–4, Unit 11).
- If you are in a residential unit shout for help and call a senior member of staff.
- If you are feeding a person in their own homes and you need support dial 999 or 112 (if using a mobile phone) and call for help.
- If the person refuses the food or drink, always respect their wishes and report the matter to a senior member of staff, who will then discuss the matter with an appropriate person, e.g. a doctor or nurse.

## How do you balance diets for different groups of service users?

A balanced diet is one that matches food intake with nutritional needs. However, it is not possible to specify a single diet that will provide for the needs of all people.

### Children

Children have a range of dietary requirements. If we ignore infants, who obtain their balanced diet from breast milk or formula baby milk, it is still clear that requirements change between the ages of 1 year and 8 years.

Protein requirements

Children grow rapidly in the first three years of life and then slow down. This is reflected in protein intake. Energy requirements in part reflect this growth, but are also affected by changes in physical activity.

A 1-year-old child may be just starting to walk, while an 8-year-old is likely to be moving about a lot more. The 8-year-old needs more energy in the diet to support this increased activity. Balancing this, a 1-year-old child loses heat faster than an 8-year-old. This is because of the younger child's size. In the small child, there is a large area of skin in relation to body weight. Heat does not have to travel far before it reaches the skin and is lost to the air. So, relatively more energy from food is needed to keep a 1-year-old warm compared to an 8-year-old.

### Vitamin requirements

These are fairly constant throughout childhood or reflect growth rates. The exception is the recommended intake of vitamin D for under-5s which is significantly higher than for older children. This is in part because of the increased rate of bone growth in under-5s, but is also to prevent rickets.

## Adolescence

### Protein requirements

The period of puberty is a time of rapid growth and great physical activity. These are reflected in increased requirements for protein and energy.

### Mineral requirements

Menarche, the first menstrual flow, is the start of a cycle of regular loss of blood. Iron is a key component of blood and so women have an increased requirement for iron in the diet compared with men, until menstruation ceases during the menopause.

## Adulthood

Throughout adulthood, differences in dietary requirements are largely related to physical activity and differences in size. If you carry out the calculations for different nutrient requirements per kilogram of body weight you will find that there is very little difference between men and women. The differences in the daily requirements are related to the fact that the average adult woman is smaller than the average adult man.

To a lesser extent, there are sex differences with regard to requirements for specific nutrients. The male hormone testosterone affects protein requirements and so men require slightly more protein than women for equivalent physically active lifestyles. As we have already mentioned, women have a greater requirement for iron.

## Pregnant women

It is often said that a pregnant woman needs to eat for two. This may be true, but in the early stages of pregnancy the growing foetus is so small that its requirements are very small. What is important is for the woman to eat a balanced diet, avoiding some of dangers associated with alcohol, drugs and smoking.

As the foetus grows, there are increased requirements for nutrients – for both the mother's needs and those of the growing baby. Protein is required for growth of the foetus. Energy is required by the foetus as well as the mother, who is using more energy than normal because of the extra weight she is carrying. Towards the end of pregnancy the woman is carrying extra weight equivalent to several bags of flour.

Vitamin and mineral requirements increase to provide for the growing foetus:

- Calcium levels in the diet need to increase to provide for the developing skeleton and also for the growth of the mother's skeleton to cope with the increased weight
- Iron requirements increase as the foetal blood forms with its need for iron.

Pregnancy is a time when a woman becomes slightly anaemic (reduced iron levels in the blood). This is natural and allows the foetus to obtain oxygen more easily. It is important not to try to correct this mild anaemia with too much iron as this can damage the foetus.

### Older people

As people get older they tend to become less physically active. This is reflected in a reduced energy requirement. Growth ceases and repair processes become slower and less efficient with age. The protein requirement in the diet reflects this.

There is good evidence that levels of calcium and vitamin D need to be increased to prevent or delay the process of calcium loss from the bones. This particularly affects women after the menopause, but it also affects men.

### Religious and cultural factors

It is only possible here to touch briefly upon some issues relating to diet in religion and culture. It is important that you recognise this and use this account only as a guideline if you are planning a diet for someone from a cultural or religious group other than your own. (If you are planning to do this, then it is important to ask about foods that should not be eaten.)

Some people will refuse to eat specific foods because of their religious beliefs. They may also require that the food that they eat is prepared in a special way. Neither orthodox Muslims nor Jews will eat pork. Both groups also require that their meat comes from animals that have been slaughtered and butchered in particular ways. These restrictions present few problems in providing a balanced diet, as the nutrients required can be provided from other sources.

Orthodox Jews also have dietary restrictions on combinations of food served in a meal. It is not acceptable to serve meat in a meal that also contains milk products. Therefore, roast beef and Yorkshire pudding (which is made from a batter containing milk) is clearly unacceptable, as would be a meal containing meat and a final course of cheese and biscuits or coffee with milk. Again, awareness of this enables well-balanced diets to be drawn up.

### Availability of food and cost of food – choice

The cost of food can have seasonal variations. More important here is a person's ability to buy the right food to produce a balanced diet. People living on low incomes or on benefits may struggle to provide a balanced diet from their available income.

There are regular articles in the press from people suggesting that it is possible to provide a balanced diet on a low income. This may be true, but the choice of foods is limited and the diet, while nutritious, could become boring and monotonous.

## How do you prepare meals hygienically?

When preparing food you must keep hygiene in mind. You must ensure that all work surfaces and equipment are clean before and after use. Good hygienic practices will make for a more pleasing workplace and will reduce the risk of infections spreading. In your work placement, you should read the basic guidelines relating to hygiene and safety rules that must be enforced.

### Hygiene

The most important thing is to wash your hands in warm water with soap before touching food.

- Wash after touching raw foods and before touching ready-to-eat foods.
- Wipe your hands on a separate kitchen towel.
- Bleach disinfect kitchen cloths often.
- Always wear protective clothing when working in the kitchen.
- Make sure that jewellery and hair are not likely to get into food.
- Cover cuts and grazes.
- Clean up spilt food straight away.
- Avoid cross-contamination of raw and cooked foods by preparing them on separate surfaces and washing hands and equipment after use.

## Serving a main course to a service user

### *Serving simple meals*

Some service users will have difficulties when eating or drinking because of their disability or illness. However, not all people with disabilities or illness will need help with eating or drinking. People react to their situation differently. Some may need support, others may not. Never impose help or support on a person: it is important that you empower them by first finding out if they require any assistance.

### *Serving meals and drinks to a group of older people with disabilities*

Refer to the section on care planning earlier in this chapter. Assess the needs of the service users to find out:

- How much they can do for themselves?
- Any special diets including cultural and religious factors?
- Likes, dislikes and choices.

Plan exactly what you are going to do. Prepare:

- Set the tables so that they look attractive – don't forget salt, pepper and sauces
- Set out specially adapted cutlery if required
- Have a jug of water or other drinks with glasses or special feeding cups
- A few small flowers look very nice
- Have napkins and possibly special bibs to protect clothing from food
- Make sure the seating arrangements are appropriate – perhaps some service users will come to the table in wheelchairs or may need to sit in a specially adapted chair. The height of the table and the space available must be considered.

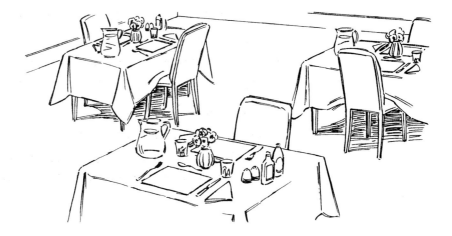

Carry out the task:

- Make sure that everyone has had the opportunity to go to the lavatory and to wash their hands
- Make sure they are comfortably seated in a place where they like to sit
- Serve the food and drink, making sure that carers are available to assist service users who are not able to feed themselves.

About the food – food and drink should:

- Take into account the dietary needs, culture and religion of the service user
- Look appetising
- Smell good
- Taste good
- Be served at the right temperature
- Be in the right quantity for the particular service user.

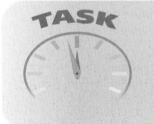

## TASK

### Diet in different cultures

Find out about a diet from a different culture.

Write up your findings.

### Hints on how to feed service users who are unable to feed themselves

You may be able to observe this in your work placement.

- Make sure the service user is seated comfortably
- Have any specialist eating aids ready
- Describe the food
- Protect clothing with bib or napkin
- Check the food temperature
- Place small amounts of food on the fork or spoon and place very gently in the mouth
- Allow plenty of time to chew and swallow
- Offer drinks during the meal
- Make the meal an enjoyable social experience.

### Safety

- Be aware of the service user's ability to chew and swallow
- Choking is a hazard

- Check the temperature of food and drinks
- Always supervise
- Observe food hygiene rules.

### Actions to take if feeding goes wrong

Sometime something goes wrong when a service user is having a meal. They may:

- Choke or cough
- Vomit.

If they have an allergic reaction to any item in the meal they might show the following symptoms:

- Their face or mouth may swell up
- They may get cramps in their muscles
- They may develop a skin rash.

If a service user shows any of these responses to a meal you must report the matter to your supervisor, who will contact a doctor immediately.

## TASK

### Serving a meal to a service user

Give one example of how you would use your skills to support a service user to choose an appropriate meal.

You will be observed demonstrating how to prepare and serve a meal to a service user and giving examples of what to do if feeding goes wrong. You must perform these tasks independently, confidently and competently.

You should also keep a logbook, which shows the theory reasons for the actions you have taken.

## AO6  Evaluate the success of the practical care provided

The process of assessment and evaluation of the practical care that you give service users enables you to evaluate and appraise the quality of the care that you have given. Evaluation means judging the worth to the service user and the quality of the practical care offered. In the light of what you find changes can be made to the care that you give.

It is very important that you evaluate how effective the practical care that you have provided is. For example is the walking aid helping the service user to be more mobile; do they need a different one? Is the diet that has been agreed with the service user providing the nutrients – or perhaps the diet was provided so that they could lose weight?

No service user's condition will remain static. They may improve and not need the support, they may deteriorate and need a different type of support, or – also important – their attitude to the support may change.

If the service user's condition remains the same, the support may need to be reviewed to see if it has to be increased or reduced. The aid the service user is using (wheelchair, hoist, etc.) may have deteriorated with use and need servicing.

If the service user's condition has deteriorated or improved then you will need to bring together all the people (nurses, carers, GPs, etc.) who made the initial decision to offer the support to review the services user's condition and the suitability of the practical support.

### Things to look for when evaluating the support

- The aim of the support.
- What was the original reason that the practical support was offered?
    - Was it short-term support? For example, were meals offered only while the service user's carer was away on holiday? Were aids to daily living offered because an elderly person had broken his/her arm and needed adapted aids for a short period?
    - Was it long- term support? For example a service user who has chronic arthritis in his/her knees and can't walk needs a wheelchair. Are they using it properly? Would a different type of chair be more appropriate?

### How do you evaluate practical care?

Example of a practical care task – serving a meal

Questions to ask yourself:

- Did you apply the care values when offering the service?
    - Did you discuss the service with the service user?
    - Did you consider their views/special requests/diet, etc?
    - Did you consider the culture or religion of the service user?
- Did you present a meal that met the nutritional requirements of the service user, if it did not why?
- Did you present the meal in a visually pleasing manner?
- Was the service user able to eat the food with the utensils provided?
- Did the service user need specially adapted knives, forks, etc?
- Did you allow the service user enough time to finish their meal?
- Have you asked the service user if they enjoyed the meal?
- Did you make arrangements to take the service user's comments into account when preparing their next meal?

When you have all the answers to these questions, would you do the same thing next time? If not, what would you do differently, how and why?

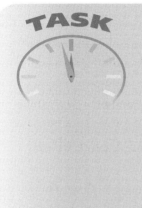

## Evaluate the effectiveness of the practical care you have provided

Choose one service user whom you have supported with practical care. Evaluate the success of this support in terms of

1. The skills you used
2. The qualities you used
3. The aim of the support
4. The objectives of the support
5. How you achieved the outcomes of the support
6. The time you allocated to the tasks
7. The improvement in the service user's well-being.

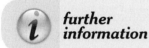

Bell L (1999) *Care Fully. A Handbook for Home Care Assistants*. Age Concern, London

Clarke L (2000) *Health and Social Care for Intermediate GNVQ*. Nelson Thornes, Cheltenham

Clarke L (2002) *Health and Social Care GCSE*. Nelson Thornes, Cheltenham

Clarke L, White M and Rowell K (2002) *An Entry Level Course in Caring*. Nelson Thornes, Cheltenham

Green S (2002) *BTEC National Early Years*. Nelson Thornes, Cheltenham

Nolan Y (1998) *Care. NVQ Level 2 Student Handbook*. Heinemann, Oxford

Nolan Y (2003) *S/NVQ Level 3 Promoting Independence*. Heinemann, Oxford

Worsley I (1999) *Taking Good Care. A Handbook for Home Care Assistants*. Age Concern, London

# Summary

- Carers should always work towards creating equality, dignity and respect for all service users. By listening to them and not labelling or talking down to them, carers will empower service users to keep as much control of their lives as possible.

- A whole range of skills is needed to ensure effective practical caring. These include interpersonal skills, patience, observation and listening.

- There are a variety of practical ways to help service users when choosing appropriate clothing and when dressing. Appropriate aids should be used if the service user agrees.

- Appropriate mobility aids can be used according to the level of help required. Assessments should always be made first by an occupational therapist or physiotherapist. Support can also be offered from bodies such as local Social Services departments or voluntary organisations.

- Understanding the components of a balanced diet is the key to being able to help service users choose a healthy diet appropriate to their needs.

- Continuing to ask questions to evaluate the effectiveness of practical care offered to a service user is very important. Is their mobility aid still appropriate? Can they now use a walking stick instead of a Zimmer frame? Was the support offered only for the short term?

# Hygiene and safety in care settings

**4**

## To complete this unit you will need to:

- Describe the risk of the spread of infection in a care setting
- Describe the measures needed to prevent the spread of infection
- Recognise basic food hygiene practices required in a care setting
- Identify basic hazards and describe ways of reducing risks in care settings
- Investigate safety and security measures required in care settings
- Understand how chemicals, including drugs, may be kept safely in care setting

**AO1** Describe the risk of the spread of infection in a care setting

Infections are caused by *microbes* (small living organisms or microorganisms). These are so small that we need a microscope to see them.

The main groups of microbes involved in infections are:

- **Bacteria** – for example tuberculosis, cholera
- **Viruses** – for example measles, influenza
- **Fungi** – for example ringworm, athlete's foot.

When a person becomes contaminated by one of these organisms, they are said to be infected.

Micro-organisms multiply very quickly under conditions of moisture, warmth and a food supply. In these conditions, they reproduce by splitting in half every 20 minutes. One or two germs could, therefore, multiply into millions in a few days.

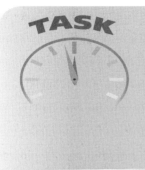

## TASK

### Multiplication of microbes

A care worker leaves a dish of chicken curry on the work surface overnight. There is one single bacterium in the chicken curry. Work out how many bacteria there will be in a few hours

| | | |
|---|---|---|
| 6.00 – 1 bacterium | 8.20 – 128 | 10.40 – |
| 6.20 – 2 bacteria | 8.40 – | 11.00 – |
| 6.40 – 4 | 9.00 – | 11.20 – |
| 7.00 – 8 | 9.20 – | 11.40 – |
| 7.20 – 16 | 9.40 – | 12.00 – |
| 7.40 – 32 | 10.00 – | |
| 8.00 – 64 | 10.20 – | |

Total number of germs produced in 6 hours =

Infection may occur in a number of different ways:

- By droplets or dust in the air
- By skin and mucous membranes
- By wounds
- By food and drink
- By soil or animals
- By infected articles.

## Risk to self and others

Prevention and control of infection are important considerations in all the care environments.

There are lots of opportunities for exposure to a wide range of germs that can carry the risk of harm and disease to both carer and service users.

### Food poisoning

Food poisoning may occur after eating contaminated or poisonous foods. The illness usually involves some or all of the following symptoms:

- Vomiting
- Diarrhoea
- Abdominal pain
- Fever (high temperature).

Table 4.1 lists the most common type of food poisoning and their causes.

*Table 4.1  Causes of food poisoning*

| Food poisoning microbe | Where found | How spread |
|---|---|---|
| *Salmonella* | Raw meat<br>Poultry<br>Eggs<br>Unwashed vegetables<br>Made-up raw foods, e.g. sausages | From food to hands<br>Contaminated food |
| *Staphylococcus aureus* | Skin<br>Nose<br>Throat<br>Boils<br>Cuts | By contaminated hands directly on to cooked food |
| *Campylobacter* | Birds<br>Dogs<br>Untreated milk<br>Poultry<br>Meat | Bird-pecked milk<br>Careless handling of meat<br>Hands |
| *Listeria* | Humans<br>Insects<br>Animals<br>Soil<br>Water | Contamination of cooked food by raw products, e.g. mayonnaise<br>Contamination of food by dust, insects, animals |
| *Escherichia coli* (*E. coli*) | Gut of man and animals<br>Soil<br>Water | Contaminated meat<br>Poor personal hygiene |

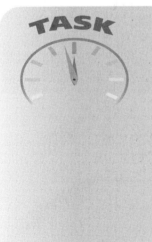

## TASK

## Causes of food poisoning

Identify the type of food poisoning most likely to occur from the following situations/conditions:

| Source/method of contamination | Food poisoning type |
|---|---|
| Drinking bird-pecked milk | |
| Eating cooked food contaminated by raw products, e.g. mayonnaise, which uses raw eggs | |
| Eating beefburgers that are not properly cooked | |

## Infectious diseases

Children can be prone to infection because their immune system is not yet fully developed.

Table 4.2 lists some of the main childhood infectious diseases.

*Table 4.2   Childhood infectious diseases*

| Bacterial infections | Viral infections |
|---|---|
| Whooping cough | German measles |
| Diphtheria | Chicken pox |
| Tuberculosis (TB) | Mumps |
| | Measles |
| | Polio |

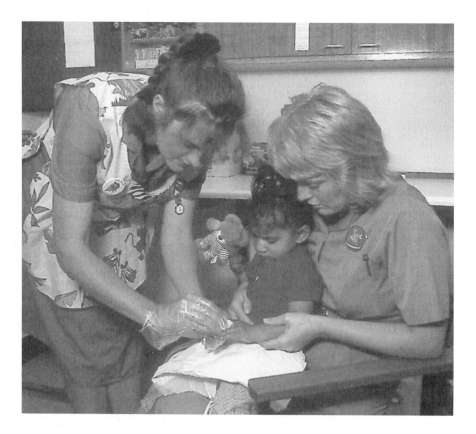

Vaccination is available to protect children from the following diseases:

- Measles
- Mumps
- Polio
- Whooping cough
- Diphtheria
- German measles
- TB.

Care service users and care workers may also be exposed to infectious diseases; these include the following.

### Methicillin-resistant Staphylococcus aureus (MRSA)

This is often referred to as a 'superbug' as it is very resistant to treatment. MRSA is usually contracted in hospital or other medical establishments. It is very important to maintain stringent cleaning and disinfecting processes as those people in hospital are already weakened by illness or surgery and will be more vulnerable to infection as a result.

### Hepatitis A

This is an infection caught by eating or drinking something that has been contaminated by infected faeces (human waste). Food prepared or washed in infected water can also spread the disease.

It is the most common cause of liver disease in the UK. The incubation period, before symptoms develop, can be between 2 and 6 weeks. Sometimes jaundice can occur. This when the liver does not function properly and the skin and whites of the eyes can become yellow. It is important to prevent dehydration by supplying regular drinks. Recovery usually takes a few weeks. In some cases, hospitalisation may be necessary.

### Hepatitis B and C

Hepatitis B is an infection carried in blood and body fluids. Hepatitis B is the only blood-borne virus for which there is a vaccine. Most employers in care settings offer this vaccine to employees as a routine precaution. It does not protect against human immunodeficiency virus (HIV) or hepatitis C. HIV and hepatitis C can be transmitted by unprotected sexual intercourse with an infected person or by inoculation with infected blood or sharing infected needles.

### The main routes of infection

Microorganisms can enter the body through:

- **The respiratory route** – this means by breathing through the nose and mouth
- **The digestive route** – through the mouth by swallowing
- **Blood** – via cuts and grazes.

**AO2**  # Describe the measures needed to prevent the spread of infection

### Basic procedures

Good standards of personal hygiene are essential to ensure the health, safety and welfare of service users and staff. Poor personal hygiene causes the spread of more diseases than anything else. The common cold and influenza (flu) are spread by droplets coughed or sneezed out by an infected person. They are also breathed out but do not spread so far.

### Cleanliness

Care workers need to ensure a high standard of personal hygiene. The skin has pores that need to be kept clean as the body rids itself of grease and sweat. If skin is left unwashed then the smell is obvious. Extra care must be given to areas where sweat is trapped in the folds of the skin. Regular washing or showering will help prevent build-up of dirt and sweat and regular use of deodorants and antiperspirants helps to prevent build-up of stale smells and keeps the person feeling fresh. Care staff are also aware of the need to:

- Use handkerchiefs – preferably disposable, as a single cough or sneeze will be hazardous to others
- Cover cuts and grazes with coloured waterproof dressings before starting work and change the dressing frequently. Use brightly coloured wound dressings that are easy to spot if they come off.
- Keep nails short and well scrubbed
- Not use nail varnish as it can become chipped and harbour bacteria.

### Dress

- Clothing needs to be regularly laundered to the correct temperature to ensure cleanliness (at least 60°C wash)
- In some care settings where uniforms are worn, special accommodation is provided for clothing that is worn at work
- Always wear protective clothing in kitchen areas
- Remove protective clothing if you leave the premises, e.g. during your lunch break
- Do not travel to your place of work in protective clothing
- Do not wear jewellery
- There may be restrictions about carrying things in your pocket that could cause injury, e.g. scissors, pen.

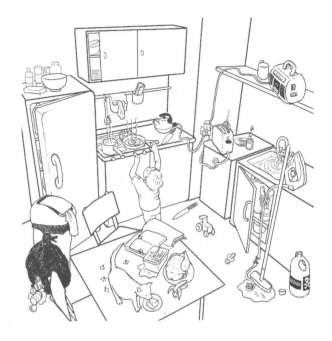

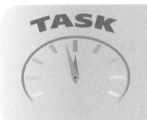

## Hygiene

Look at the kitchen in the illustration. List and explain all the unhygienic practices you can see.

### *Protective clothing*

Some personal care procedures, e.g. helping service users to feed themselves, may require the care worker to use protective clothing. Protective clothing can include:

- Overalls
- Latex-free gloves and disposable aprons for high-risk, messy activities such as changing incontinence pads or collecting a blood sample
- Goggles – safe, suitable and comfortable, cleaned and stored safely on the premises
- Masks
- Gowns.

### *Hand washing*

- Wash hands frequently in running water
- Wipe hands on separate towels, preferably disposable towels. Regularly launder and disinfect towels

- It is a good practice to use a bactericidal detergent from a dispenser. An antiseptic rub, applied to clean hands, provides an alternative to bactericidal soap
- Drying facilities may include disposable paper, warm air dryers, roller paper cabinet towels, washable fabric roller
- Where nail brushes are provided, they must be kept clean
- It is good practice to have signs to identify 'hand wash' basins.

### Hair care

Some people need to wash their hair more frequently than others because their skin and scalp are naturally more oily. Things like taking exercise, cooking or being in a smoky environment can also affect how often the hair needs washing. In some care settings it is good practice to tie long hair back and staff working in kitchen areas will need to wear protective hats. Hair can spread infection and also, if it is loose, it could become entangled in equipment and cause injury.

### Footwear

Some general guidelines include:

- Keep toe-nails short and remove hard skin
- See a doctor or chiropodist for anything more serious, such as athlete's foot, bunions or corns
- Wear comfortable shoes with a low heel to prevent injury to self and others – slipping on floors, for example, is the main cause of accidents in kitchens and care homes
- Footwear should be cleaned regularly as bacteria can be easily transported into care settings
- Do not wear open-toed shoes.

### Oral hygiene

Clean teeth mean healthy teeth and less chance of bad breath. Every time you eat, a harmful substance called plaque starts to build up on your teeth. Teeth should be cleaned at least twice a day – in the morning and before going to bed. Particular attention needs to be paid to the gum line. Anti-bactericidal mouth washes can help to maintain oral hygiene. A visit to the dentist every 6 months is usually recommended.

## Conditions that require reporting when working in care settings

The Reporting of Injuries, Diseases and Danger Occurrences Regulations 1995 (RIDDOR) require employers and others to report certain types of injury, occupational ill-health and dangerous occurrences that can happen as a result of work. These can include the following categories:

- Poisoning – e.g. by contact with chemicals, food poisoning
- Skin diseases – e.g. dermatitis
- Lung disease – e.g. asthma as a result of working with dangerous substances
- Infectious diseases – e.g. hepatitis
- Musculoskeletal disorders e.g. repetitive strain injury (RSI).

Records must be kept in care settings, available for inspection, of any reportable diseases. Certain diseases are termed 'notifiable'. This means that the relevant medical authorities must be notified immediately if they occur, so that carers, service users and the wider community can be alerted and protected. Major notifiable diseases include food poisoning, measles, whooping cough and meningitis.

## Universal precautions

- Wash hands before and after contact with service users
- Wash hands before and after using latex-free gloves
- Use brightly coloured waterproof dressings to cover any cuts, grazes or wounds
- Always wear gloves when dealing with blood or other body fluids
- Be very careful in handling and disposing of sharps, including scalpels, scissors and needles
- Do not wear open footwear where blood or other body fluids may be spilt or where sharp instruments are used
- Spillage involving blood or bodily fluid should be cleaned up promptly and the area disinfected
- Follow procedures for the safe disposal of any contaminated clinical waste
- Wear protective eyegear when exposed to blood and body fluids. Treat accidental exposure with eye wash.

All care settings will have in place infection control policies, which cover all aspects of care practice.

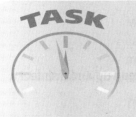

## TASK

## Designing a hygiene instructions booklet

You are a care worker in charge of a team of care assistants. Sunil has joined your team and he is having difficulty understanding written instructions because English is his second language.

Design a booklet of pictorial instructions that will help Sunil understand about the universal hygiene precautions needed in a care setting.

of hazardous substances in the workplace. All care settings must have an up-to-date COSHH file listing all the hazardous substances stored and used on their premises.

The file must:

- Identify and name the hazardous substance
- State where each hazardous substance is kept
- State what the labels are
- Describe the effects of the substances
- State the outside limits within which it is safe to be exposed to the substance
- Describe how to deal with an emergency.

## Locations

In any building, home or workplace, some locations are potentially more hazardous than others. More accidents happen in kitchens, bathrooms and stairs than in any other part of the care setting. Slips are the main cause of accidents in kitchens. Electrical equipment in all areas should be checked regularly.

### Kitchen

- It is important that the layout of the kitchen is well planned. There should always be enough room for the safe preparation and serving of food
- Ventilation is also very important, as kitchens can become very hot and this can lead to moisture forming on all surfaces, creating slippery floors
- Care should be taken when installing equipment – for example, a deep fat frier should not be placed next to a sink
- All surfaces must be easy to clean and maintain
- If pesticides are used they must be approved for use in the kitchen
- Food must be stored correctly at correct temperatures
- Staff must be trained in kitchen hygiene and use of equipment
- Animals must not be allowed in the kitchen area.

### Bathrooms

- Thermostatic mixing valves must be fitted to prevent scalding
- Adequate training and supervision must be given to ensure that staff involved in bathing service users understand the risks and precautions
- Carers must take into account the vulnerability of the service user when meeting their personal hygiene needs. An assessment of the service user's capabilities should be carried out regularly to determine the level of support needed, particularly with reference to assistive devices

- No locks on doors
- Ensure that bath and shower both have non-slip mats
- Grab rails should always be in place
- Carers should be aware that bath oils can also increase the risk of slipping
- All bathing equipment and toiletries should be within easy reach
- The bathroom should be warm and well ventilated.

### Stairs

- The stairs should be well lit
- Stair coverings should be in good condition and securely fastened
- There should be no obstructions
- Smoke alarms should be fitted at every level.

### Community rooms

- Communal space should be available to allow service users access to social, cultural and religious activities
- Non-slip flooring
- Well lit – to allow for reading and other activities
- No trailing flexes on televisions or electrical appliances
- Exits and entrances should not be blocked or obstructed
- Heating should meet the relevant environmental health and safety requirements and the needs of individual service users.

### Bedrooms

- Service users should have safe, comfortable bed rooms, with their own possessions around them
- There should be two double electric sockets, and they should be easily accessible
- Beds should be at a suitable, safe height for the service user
- Service users should have a key unless their risk assessment suggests otherwise
- Rooms are centrally heated but controlled in the service user's own room
- Emergency lighting is provided throughout the care setting
- It is useful to have an emergency alarm installed in each room
- A no-smoking policy should be enforced in bed rooms.

### Entrance halls

- Closed-circuit TV (CCTV) coverage for security purposes

- Entrances should be wide enough to accommodate wheelchairs and stretchers
- Well lit
- Glazing materials appropriate
- Floor coverings should be non-slip
- Furniture and equipment should be kept tidy, to avoid the risk of injury
- Security code lock on the door to prevent vulnerable service users leaving the building unaccompanied.

## Reducing risks

### Safety surveys/audits

Managing health and safety is a legal duty under the management of Health and Safety at Work Regulations 1992. The regulations require health and safety to be managed by having effective health and safety arrangements. Health and safety needs must be assessed, planned for, organised, controlled, monitored and reviewed. Regular safety surveys are an essential part of this process.

Risk assessment is a careful identification and examination of what could cause harm to people. Precautions and safety measures can then be decided upon aimed at minimising the risks. The main aim of safety surveys or risk assessment is to make sure that no one gets hurt or becomes ill as a result of a potential hazard.

The safety survey must be regularly updated and the document available for inspection.

### Staff training

A competent person or persons must be appointed to assist with health and safety in the care setting. It is also important that health and safety training and information is made available to all staff, including night staff. Supervision must also be provided where appropriate.

Under the Health and Safety (First Aid) Regulations 1981 there should be at least one appointed person who will take charge in an emergency situation. It is recommended that an appointed person should have up to date emergency first aid training. Staff will also require training on moving and handling, first aid and the control of infection.

It is a key duty of health and safety legislation that staff are provided with information, instruction and training.

### Safety features

A basic function of all care organisations is to provide a safe and controlled environment for staff, service users and visitors. The wide-ranging nature of care organisations means that each organisation has its own particular requirements in terms of health and safety. For example, nurseries playgroups will have different requirements from a home for older Each has their own particular hazards.

### Regular checking of equipment

All equipment must be checked regularly to ensure it is in good working order. Only competent and qualified personnel must be permitted to inspect, test and maintain specific pieces of equipment. Records should be kept of all inspections.

### Following rules and regulations

All care settings will have their own rules and regulations, designed to protect the service users and care workers, which will relate to their own particular circumstances.

### Putting policies in place

Care settings will have their own policies, which will reflect current health and safety legislation. For example, all care settings will have a waste control policy, which will take into account COSHH regulations. There should also be policies reflecting the centre's approach to moving and handling, first aid, food hygiene, health and safety and the reporting of injuries and dangerous occurrences.

### Providing safety warnings/notices

Safety signs communicate information, such as warning of a hazard – for example a slippery floor – or showing the way to a fire exit.

Regulations specify certain types to be used that are instantly recognisable by everyone. Employers must explain the meaning of signs and ensure that everyone understands what action should be taken. Safety signs must be kept in good condition.

### Correct storage of hazardous substances

It is essential to identify any harmful substances. Substances must be stored in their original containers and have safety labels and safety information clearly displayed. If dangerous chemicals have to be decanted, they should be poured into containers approved by the manufacturer and labelled appropriately. Service users have died after mistaking cleaning fluids for a drink.

## Benefits of reducing risks: to service users and staff

Accidents and illness cause a great deal of pain and suffering for individuals as well as worry and financial difficulty for families. Employers have to provide temporary cover during staff absence and this can be costly. Most people spend a considerable amount of their time at work and they do not expect their health to be damaged by work-related injury.

It is also important that carers reduce the risks to service users. To do this the workplace must be free of any risk that could put a service user at risk. It is the carer's role to try and identify and reduce potential risks to service users. If you believe that you have found a potential risk that the employer has no knowledge of you must inform them.

Service users can be put at risk by many things. Physical risks could include a slippery floor, very hot water and unlocked medicine cabinets. Other risks can be subtler, for example, has the establishment a policy on admitting strangers into the home? Service users can also be at risk from the abusive or bullying behaviour from other service users or staff.

## AO5 Investigate safety and security measures required in care settings

### Fire hazards

The Fire Precautions Act 1971 is the main law controlling fire safety. It requires certain types of establishment – such as homes for older people, hospitals, schools, colleges and hotels – to apply for a fire certificate from the fire service. This certificate must be obtained before the establishment can operate.

It is the management's responsibility to provide:

- Adequate routes for escape
- A way of giving fire warning
- Fire-fighting equipment

*A fire action notice*

> ### Maryland Home for Elderly People
> **FIRE RULES**
>
> If you discover a fire:
>
> **Raise the alarm** by operating the nearest fire alarm and proceed to the assembly point at the nearest exit (Outside the Day Room Exit).
>
> **Please go along the corridor through the Day Room and out through the double-opening patio doors.**
>
> **Close the door of your room** as you leave and any others you may use.
>
> **Do Not:**
> - use lifts as a means of escape
> - shout or run
>
> **Study this notice** carefully so that you will know what to do in an emergency.
>
> **Do not re-enter the building until told to do so by an appropriate person.**

- Written instructions for clients, workers and visitors displayed in prominent positions
- Instructions and training for staff
- Fire procedures and drills.

*The different types of fire extinguisher*

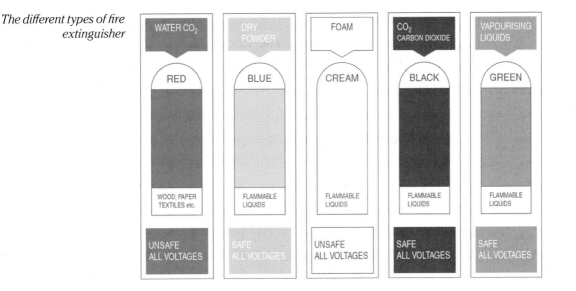

## Firefighting

- Are portable fire extinguishers and/or hose reels provided in clearly visible and readily accessible places throughout the premises?
- Are they maintained at regular intervals?
- Are staff familiar with their use?

## What should you do if you discover a fire?

You should notify a senior member of staff who should:

- Ensure that the fire service has been called
- Go to the scene of the fire and supervise the fire fighting until the fire service arrives
- Clear everyone, except those actually engaged in the fire fighting, from the immediate vicinity of the fire
- Order the evacuation of the building as soon as it becomes apparent that fire or smoke is spreading – do not wait until the fire is out of control
- Take a roll call of all staff and residents or clients when the premises have been evacuated (a list of absentees from the building should be available)
- **Do not use lifts**.

Instructions should be given to caretakers and maintenance staff, setting out the action they should take in the event of fire. This should include:

- Bringing all lifts to ground level and stopping them
- Shutting down all services not essential to the escape of occupants or likely to be required by the fire brigade.

Lighting should be left on.

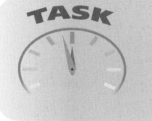

## TASK

### Fire evacuation procedures

Find out what the fire evacuation procedure is in your school, college or work placement. Explain this procedure clearly to your colleagues.

## Security of buildings

It is important that care service users feel safe and secure in their care setting. The following measures are a guide to assessing the level of security that could be in place to protect service users, staff, visitors and service personnel.

How to prevent access of unwanted callers:

- Doors to the building have an entry phone system whereby callers announce their presence and give their personal details, the nature of their visit and, where necessary, the organisation they represent
- Staff at reception screen callers upon arrival
- Service users are able to choose whom they can see and do not see, unless they have seriously diminished responsibility (e.g. advanced dementia), in which case responsibility falls to the key worker
- The wishes of service users with regard to visitors must be adhered to
- There may be restraining orders on certain individuals connected with service users. These must be strictly adhered to
- Designated personnel deal with security at night
- Doors automatically close and lock when anyone leaves the building.

The building and the grounds surrounding it must also be assessed in terms of security. Most care settings have some or all of the following in place:

- CCTV cameras at main entrance and exit points – these must be loaded with videotape
- The area surrounding the building illuminated at night
- The perimeter area securely cordoned off using fences or shrubs that deter unwanted callers

- Security alarm systems in place – with a direct line to the local police station
- Security patrols by hired contractors with professional expertise
- Regular police sweep of the area by patrol areas
- Windows double glazed to a high standard and securely locked.

### Keys

- Only authorised personnel should have access to keys
- Duplicates should be available in case of emergencies.

### Unaccompanied packages

There is a heightened awareness in today's world about the possible dangers posed by unaccompanied packages.

- Care centres need to have a policy in place and all staff need to be aware of this policy
- Do not touch or handle
- Alert staff
- Evacuate the building if the package is considered to be suspicious
- Seek advice from the police
- Return to the premises after the 'all-clear' has been given.

## Security of people

### Staff

- There should be up-to-date staff photographs on display
- Staff should wear identity cards with their photograph on
- Staff should use swipe cards for entry to the building or to different areas.

### Visitors

- Temporary visitors' badges must be pinned on to clothing and be clearly visible
- Visitors book – visitors must write down name, reason for visit, organisation, time of arrival, time of departure
- Visitors have to be buzzed out and must hand their badges back into main reception.

### Service personnel

A wide variety of people visit care centres. These can include couriers, emergency services, kitchen and stores delivery, laundry services and waste disposal teams. It is important to include them in your risk assessment. Some procedures to follow include:

- All deliveries and transactions to be signed for and records kept
- Check identification cards
- Some service personnel visits will be scheduled and therefore expected.

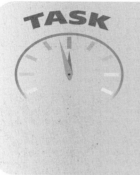

## Security procedures

Visit a care centre near you. Ask to see their risk assessment policy about security.

Check the school or college you study in. What security measures are in place?

Do you feel they are adequate?

# Understand how chemicals, including drugs, may be kept safely in care settings

The Control of Substances Hazardous to Health Regulations 1999 (COSHH) outline the essential requirements and a sensible approach for the control of hazardous substances.

Hazardous substances used in care settings include some cleaning materials, disinfectants and microorganisms (associated with clinical waste or soiled laundry). Drugs and medicines are also classed as hazardous.

## The Control of Substances Hazardous to Health Regulations 1988

These regulations lay down the essential requirements and a sensible step-by-step approach for the control of hazardous substances, such as poisons, gas or chemicals, and for protecting people who are exposed to them.

What is a substance hazardous to health? Some substances used by carers are obviously dangerous. Others are not obviously hazardous until they are misused or used in the wrong place. For example, a bottle of bleach is not in itself harmful but if it is left in a place where confused people or children could drink it, it would then become a hazard. Many substances can therefore be a hazard in one situation and not in another.

There is a wide range of substances capable of damaging health. Many are used for cleaning or decorating. The health of carers can be put at risk from these substances if the right precautions are not taken.

Many of these substances are labelled so that people know what they are dealing with. For example, labels indicate whether a substance is:

- Very toxic
- Toxic

*Some examples of hazard labels*

Corrosive

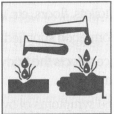

Oxidising

Toxic

Harmful irritant

Highly flammable

Explosive

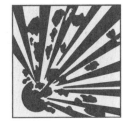

- Harmful
- Irritant
- Corrosive
- Composed of any material, mixture or compound that can harm people's health.

The possible toxic effects of chemicals are:

- Occupational dermatitis (skin disorder)
- Headaches
- Irritability
- Nausea and vomiting (sickness)
- Dizziness
- Nose and throat irritation
- Tiredness
- Sleeplessness
- Chest trouble
- Worsening of asthma (a lung condition)
- Reproductive hazards (may affect the ability to have children)
- Heart, lung, liver disease
- Kidney damage
- Cancer.

## Safe use of chemicals

Poor working practices when handling chemicals, cleaners and powders

**Describe the principles of caring for the sick child**

Sick children still have physical, intellectual, emotional and social needs; they also need to play.

## Physical needs

The child will need *warmth*, but it is also important that the room should be kept ventilated to prevent the child from becoming overheated.

*Food and drink* are also necessary. If the child is not well enough to eat, then plenty of liquids should be offered. Diluted fruit juices are ideal and will provide the child with additional vitamin C. Tempt children with small, well-presented portions of their favourite foods. Little but often is a good rule.

*Sleep* is important as it allows the body to recover from illness. Naps should be encouraged throughout the day and the child should be made comfortable and allowed to rest whenever s/he wishes.

*Hygiene* is important and the child must be kept clean and comfortable. The face should be washed when necessary as this helps to freshen up the child. The hair too should be brushed and kept tidy. Clean night clothes will also help keep the child feeling fresh. The child needs to have his/her bed re-made morning and evening, with bedding changed if necessary. The window in the room should be opened to keep the room well ventilated, which will help get rid of germs. If the child has an infectious illness then s/he should be kept away from other children.

## Safety needs

### Environmental

- Ensure bedroom is kept scrupulously clean
- Ensure carers wash their hands after going in to the patient
- Bed linen and towels must be kept separate, and washed at 60°C
- The child should use paper handkerchiefs, which can then be disposed of.

### Medical

- Ensure instructions on medicines are followed exactly
- Only medicines prescribed by a doctor should be used for children
- Medicine should not be left in the room with the child
- Report any side effects of the medicine to the doctor.

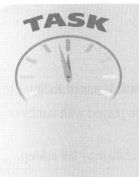

## Safety of medicines

Make a list of the medicines and tablets (e.g. cough medicines, painkillers, inhalers) that you have in your house.

Where do you keep them?

Do you finish a course of prescribed medicine?

How should you dispose of any unused medication?

### Social contact

- If the illness is infectious, the child should be isolated until there is no likelihood of passing on the infection.

### Intellectual stimulation

- Any toys used by the patient should be washed
- Games should be wiped over with a disinfectant solution
- Comics should be disposed of.

## Intellectual needs

When children are ill they often sleep for most of the day, but the carer should plan activities for when the child feels well enough to play. Activities should be short, and not too difficult to complete. When ill, children often play with toys they played with when they were younger, or revert to comfort toys such as old teddies or dolls.

## Emotional needs

When children are ill they may become more clingy than usual and need more attention from the carer. It is important that the child is reassured that they are still loved and that they will get better. Illness is worrying for anyone, but especially so for a child who is afraid and cannot express his/her feelings. Time spent with the child will make him/her feel secure and will help the recovery process.

## Social needs

If the child's illness is not infectious, and the child is well enough, friends should be encouraged to visit. This will help the child stay in touch with friends so he/she still feels part of the outside world.

## Play

Even when a child is ill play is still important. Play will help to pass the time between rests and the child will be able to use play to voice her/his concerns and worries.

mother visits the antenatal clinic (which may be held at her local health centre or hospital, depending on where she lives) first at 8–10 weeks. Further visits are then made every month up to week 28, every 2 weeks to week 36 and finally every week until delivery. Various check-ups take place, such as:

- Foetal heartbeat – checked every visit after 16 weeks
- Blood test – done at 16 weeks to check for hepatitis B and foetal abnormality
- Ultrasound scan – to check that the baby is developing correctly
- Early dating scan – done before 16 weeks to give exact age of foetus
- Anomaly scan – done around 20 weeks to check for abnormalities of limbs or internal organs. Also gives the size and sex of the foetus, the heartbeat and the position of the umbilical cord and placenta.

## Postnatal clinics

Both mother and baby are checked over at the 6-week postnatal examination. This can be carried out at a hospital or by the family GP. The baby is examined to ensure that s/he is developing normally and making healthy progress. The mother is checked to ensure that her uterus has returned to normal and that any postnatal bleeding has stopped.

## Roles of professional health workers

### General practitioner (GP)

The first person that we go to for health care within the community is the general practitioner or family doctor. GPs are qualified doctors who have undergone special training. Everyone permanently resident or working in the UK may be registered with a GP. They may select their own GP when they are over 16 years old from the list of GPs kept by the local health authority.

The first port of call for most people requiring health care is the doctor's surgery. The GP:

- Diagnoses (finds out) what is wrong with an individual
- May prescribe treatment, such as medicines, which are then obtained from a pharmacist.

GPs are specialists in general diagnosis; that is they try to find out what is wrong with you. They have a good knowledge of a broad range of types of ill-health. When they do not have the facilities or skills to diagnose or treat a patient, they refer the patient to a specialist doctor based in a hospital, for example if a person needs an operation.

Some doctors' surgeries dispense the medicines that the doctors prescribe. This usually happens in rural or remote areas where it is difficult for patients to get to a pharmacist.

It is now common for a group of GPs to work together in a local centre. Each of the doctors will have the general diagnostic skills, but each will also have a specialist interest or skill to contribute to the practice. The move towards group practices started in the 1960s. It is now also very common for a practice to be based in a health centre.

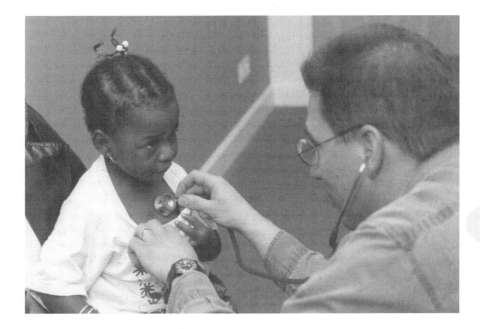

### Health visitor

As mentioned previously the health visitor is part of a health centre team. The health visitor is a qualified nurse who has gained midwifery qualifications as well as qualifications in family health and child development. As a result of this the health visitor will work with all ages in the community, from newborn babies to older people. Health visitors may run baby/toddler clinics, as well as visiting people in their own homes to offer advice and support. Health visitors will carry out child health screening until the child starts school (see below).

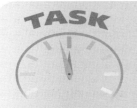

## TASK

## Monitoring child growth

Choose one of the three health professionals listed:

- GP
- Health visitor
- Paediatrician

Find out about the work involved in the job. You might even be able to interview.

From the information you have gained, write about a typical day in the professional life of your chosen person.

### Paediatricians

These are qualified doctors who have specialised in childhood illnesses. They are usually based in hospitals or clinics. They carry out medical checks on babies born in hospital and care for the health of children throughout childhood. Children with physical illnesses would be referred to a paediatrician by their GP or family doctor.

## Ways in which support is provided

### Screening

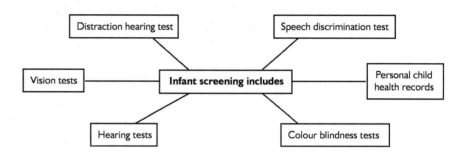

All children are checked regularly to ensure that they are growing and developing normally. Health screening is important, as any health problems can be picked up at an early age – e.g. a hearing problem that the parents may not be aware of. Centile charts are used to record the child's height, weight and, if under 1 year, head circumference. Also, the child will have a physical examination, and will be observed carrying out activities.

Below are the general guidelines for child health screening:

- **Neonatal check** – at birth by midwife and by paediatrician before baby leaves hospital

- **6 weeks** – postnatal examination of mother also carried out by GP

- **6–9 months** – carried out by health visitor and will include a hearing test. Advice will also be given on diet and hygiene, together with any other advice the mother needs

- **18–24 months** – as this is the beginning of the 'terrible twos', advice will be given on temper tantrums. Diet and potty training will also be covered by health visitor. Observation will be made of the child walking

- **36–44 months** – Health visitor will carry out this preschool check. Parents can seek any advice they require.

Once the child starts school, the school nurse will check height and weight.

Throughout the checks, if there are any problems the child will be seen by the GP on a more regular basis.

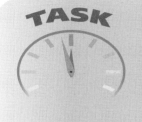

## TASK

### Monitoring child growth

Choose a 3–4-year-old child. Using the hospital or clinic baby development booklet for height/weight information, plot their progress on the appropriate centile chart.

### Medication

The family doctor will prescribe any medication needed for the baby/young child and will monitor the child's progress throughout the course. It is generally better to give a baby/young child prescribed medication rather than medication bought over the counter at a chemist.

### Personal support and advice

All the primary care team based at the family's medical centre will offer support and advice to the family of the sick child. Health visitors and GPs will offer home visits and will monitor progress.

## Hospitalisation of children

### Emotional reaction

Staying in hospital can be a very upsetting experience for children. As well as feeling ill, or suffering pain, the child will be in unfamiliar surroundings with a different bed, different food, a new routine and strange carers. Children may be afraid and feel insecure. Parents can prepare their child by discussing the hospital with them. Explaining that they will be better when they come out can also help. It is a good idea, if possible, to visit the hospital beforehand. Many hospitals offer pre-admission visits so children can see where they are to be staying, meet the staff who will care for them and see the equipment that will be used. Parental reassurance is important and children should be told that they will be missed. Parents will be allowed to visit at any time and may stay overnight. When they leave, they should tell the child when they are coming back.

### Pre-admission activities

Before the child visits the hospital it is a good idea to explain to the child about hospitals, and this can be done by:

- Encouraging the child to dress up as a doctor or nurse and act out a hospital scene.
- Telling stories.
- Using prepared books and videos about children in hospital.
- Explaining what happens in a hospital, stressing how much better the child will feel after being in hospital.

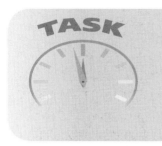

## Preparing a child for a hospital stay

In small groups, design and make a book, game or video to prepare a 6-year-old for his/her stay in hospital.

*The stay in hospital*

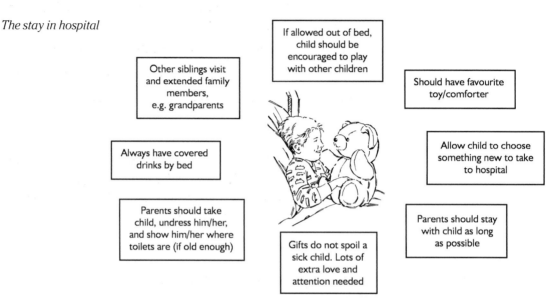

Other siblings visit and extended family members, e.g. grandparents

If allowed out of bed, child should be encouraged to play with other children

Should have favourite toy/comforter

Always have covered drinks by bed

Allow child to choose something new to take to hospital

Parents should take child, undress him/her, and show him/her where toilets are (if old enough)

Gifts do not spoil a sick child. Lots of extra love and attention needed

Parents should stay with child as long as possible

**AO4**  # Identify key signs and symptoms of common childhood illnesses and understand the care needs required

### Key signs and symptoms of a high temperature (hyperthermia)

Hyperthermia occurs when the body temperature is dangerously above normal body heat. An abnormally hot forehead may be the first indication that a child has a temperature (fever). In any infectious illness there are three stages – incubation, fever and recovery. Incubation is the stage where germs invade the body and breed rapidly. The body's response is for the immune system to produce antibodies to fight them off. The fever happens when the war between germs and antibodies is at its peak. This war produces heat, and that is why the child has a flushed face and burning skin. The body temperature rises and the child sweats. While this is a good sign that the body is gathering its defences, it is a good idea not to let the child's temperature become too high. If the child has a high temperature, s/he will be very hot, uncomfortable and irritable. In young children a very high temperature can lead to convulsions, so it is important to reduce the child's temperature.

## How to care for a child with a high temperature

- Remove any bed covering.
- Remove the child's clothing.
- Try tepid sponging if the temperature rises to 39°C or over (see below).
- After 5 minutes of tepid sponging, take child's temperature. If it has dropped to 38°C, stop sponging. If not, keep sponging for another 5 minutes, take temperature again, and repeat sponging if temperature remains higher than 38°C.
- Once the temperature drops, cover the child with a sheet.
- Watch carefully and, if the temperature rises, repeat tepid sponging.
- Call the doctor if the temperature does not drop.

### *Tepid sponging*

Half fill a bowl or bucket with tepid (lukewarm) water and place several sponges or flannels in the bowl. Wring one out slightly (it should still be dripping) and wipe over child's face and body, replacing with another when the sponge becomes warm.

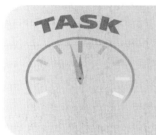

### TASK

### Reducing a child's temperature

Using ICT, design and make an informative poster to help a parent/carer reduce a child's high temperature.

## Common childhood infectious diseases

*Table 5.1 Common childhood infectious diseases*

| Disease | Caused by | Signs and symptoms | Care |
|---------|-----------|--------------------|------|
| Mumps | Virus | • Swelling of glands on either side of face below ears and beneath chin<br>• Pain when swallowing<br>• Dry mouth<br>• Fever<br>• Headache<br>Boys<br>• Painful testes<br>Girls<br>• Low abdominal back pain | 1. Check temperature to see if fever present. If there is fever, try to bring it down with tepid sponging<br>2. Give liquid food, such as milk shakes and soups<br>3. Give plenty of liquids to drink<br>4. Consult doctor to confirm mumps<br>5. Keep child at home until 5 days after swelling has gone |

▶

| | | | |
|---|---|---|---|
| Measles | Virus | • Fever (temp. can rise to 40°C<br>• Running nose<br>• Headache<br>• Dry cough<br>• Small, white spots inside mouth<br>• Small, brownish red spots, starting behind ears and spreading over body<br>• Red, sore eyes, intolerant of bright light | 1. Check temperature to see if fever present. If there is fever, try to bring it down with tepid sponging<br>2. If eyes are sore, bathe with cool water and keep in darkened room if light sensitive<br>3. Ensure child has plenty of liquids to drink<br>4. Keep child in bed until temperature comes down<br>5. Consult doctor<br>6. Do not send child back to school until rash has faded |
| Rubella | Virus | • Slightly raised temperature<br>• Enlarged, swollen glands at back of neck<br>• Tiny red spots, starting behind ears and spreading to forehead, then rest of body | 1. Inform any woman who might be pregnant and has been near the child that s/he has rubella<br>2. Keep child away from public places<br>3. If temperature is 38°C or above, offer Calpol or other paracetamol elixir |
| Whooping cough | Bacteria | • Cold symptoms of a fever, aches, pains and runny nose<br>• Excessive coughing with characteristic 'whoop' as child struggles to draw breath<br>• Coughing bout leads to vomiting<br>• Sleeplessness due to coughing | 1. If cold does not improve and cough worsens, consult doctor<br>2. If child is having coughing bout, sit him/her up and hold him/her up so he/she is leaning slightly forward. Hold bowl nearby so he/she can spit phlegm into it<br>3. Keep child calm during coughing fit, as panic will make breathlessness worse<br>4. If child vomits after coughing bout, give him/her small meals and drinks afterwards. This gives the child a better chance of keeping food down<br>5. Do not leave child alone during coughing fit<br>6. Ensure the child does not play too energetically as this will bring on coughing and leave him/her exhausted |

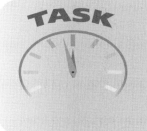

**TASK**

## Surveying views on the triple vaccine programme

Interview ten parents about their views on the MMR vaccination programme. In general, are parents in favour of the triple vaccine?

*Table 5.2  Infections of the respiratory system*

| Disease | Caused by | Signs and symptoms | Care |
|---|---|---|---|
| Common cold | Virus | • Raised temperature<br>• Sneezing<br>• Running or blocked nose<br>• Sore throat<br>• Coughing<br>• Aching muscles<br>• Irritability<br>• Catarrh | 1. Check if child has a temperature. If temperature is 38°C or above, try tepid sponging<br>2. Give child plenty to drink<br>3. Help child to blow nose properly by blowing one nostril at a time<br>4. Sprinkle camphor on bedding and/or clothing which will help child breathe easier during the night<br>5. To help sore throat, give child a hot drink of lemon juice and water before bed |
| Tonsillitis | Bacteria | • Sore throat<br>• Difficulty in swallowing<br>• Red, enlarged tonsils<br>• Temperature of over 38°C<br>• Swollen glands in neck<br>• Unpleasant breath | 1. If cold does not improve and cough worsens, consult doctor<br>2. If child is having a coughing bout, sit him/her up and hold him/her up so s/he is leaning slightly forward. Hold bowl nearby so s/he can spit phlegm into it<br>3. Keep child calm during coughing fit, as panic will make breathlessness worse<br>4. If child vomits after a coughing bout, give him/her small meals and drinks afterwards. This gives the child a better chance of keeping food down<br>5. Do not leave child alone during a coughing fit<br>6. Ensure that the child does not play too energetically, as this will bring on coughing and leave the child exhausted |

*Table 5.3  Infections of the gastrointestinal tract*

| Disease | Caused by | Signs and Symptoms | Care |
|---|---|---|---|
| Gastroenteritis | Virus<br>Bacteria | • Nausea<br>• Vomiting<br>• Diarrhoea<br>• Abdominal cramps<br>• Loss of appetite<br>• Raised temperature | 1. Stop all food, and milk, and give the child small sips of water every 15 minutes<br>2. Put the child to bed with a bowl/bucket beside the bed in case s/he vomits<br>3. Consult a doctor if the child has vomiting and diarrhoea for more than 6 hours<br>4. Be meticulous about hygiene<br>5. Do not give the child acidic drinks such as orange juice |

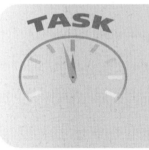

## Assessing a sick child

Jordan has a temperature of 38.5°C. He has vomited several times during the day, and has refused all food. It is now late afternoon and, although he has stopped vomiting, he is very drowsy and hard to wake.

What should Jordan's carers do?

**AO5**  **Demonstrate correct health measuring, monitoring and recording techniques**

### Measuring the pulse

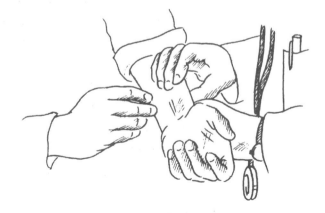

Each time the heart beats to pump blood, a wave passes along the walls of the arteries. This wave is the pulse and it can be felt at any point in the body where a large artery crosses a bone just beneath the skin. The pulse is usually counted at the radial artery in the wrist or the carotid artery in the neck. To take a pulse, the fingertips (but not the thumb tips) are placed over the site where the pulse is being taken. The beats are counted for a full minute and then recorded. Normally the rhythm is regular and the volume is sufficient to make the pulse easily felt. The three main observations which are made on the pulse are rate, rhythm and strength. The average adult pulse rate varies between 60 and 80 beats per minute, while a young baby has a heart rate of about 140 beats per minute. An increased pulse rate may indicate recent exercise, emotion, infection, blood or fluid loss, shock and heart disease.

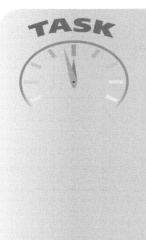

## TASK

### Measuring the pulse

Working with a partner, take his/her resting pulse. Record it. Ask your partner to walk up and down stairs twice. Take your partner's pulse again. Record it. Then get your partner to run on the spot for 30 seconds. Take his/her pulse immediately. Record it.

Resting pulse =

Walking up and down stairs =

Running on the spot =

What do the results tell you?

Repeat the exercise with your partner taking your pulse readings.

## Body mass index

We are all familiar with our own body size and shape. Looking around we can see there is an immense variation in others' sizes and shapes. We are all individuals. If, however, a person is underweight, this can be an indicator of their physical health. The body mass index is often used to measure this aspect of health. Body mass index (BMI) can be calculated by dividing a person's weight (in kilograms) by the square of their height (in metres). This can then be used as a guide to five BMI groups:

- Underweight: BMI 19.9 and below
- Normal: BMI 20–24.9
- Overweight: BMI 25–29.9
- Obese: BMI 30–39.9
- Severely obese: BMI 40 and above.

## Average or normal

It is important to remember that it is possible to be different from the average in height, weight, length, etc., but still be within normal limits.

## Weight

The average weight for a newborn baby is 3.5kg (7lb 11oz). The heaviest recorded live-born baby weighed in at 9.3kg (20lb 8oz)! Babies should be weighed regularly, as weight gain and contentment are signs that they are being fed adequately. A baby can be expected to double his/her birth weight in the first 6 months and treble it by the end of the first year.

Children (and adults) will become fat if they overeat and do not have enough exercise. They can tend to overeat if they are worried, bored or insecure. It is unwise to give a small child too many sweets or fattening foods. Excessive weight gain in the early years makes it more likely that a child will be overweight in later life.

*Table 5.4  Average weights and heights for young children*

| Age | Weight | | Height | |
|-----|--------|----|--------|----|
|     | kg | lb | cm | in |
| **Girls** | | | | |
| Birth | 3.4 | 7.5 | 53.0 | 20.9 |
| 3 months | 5.6 | 12.3 | | |
| 6 months | 6.9 | 15.2 | | |
| 9 months | 8.7 | 19.2 | | |
| 1 year | 9.7 | 21.4 | 74.2 | 29.2 |
| 2 years | 12.2 | 26.9 | 85.6 | 33.7 |
| 3 years | 14.3 | 31.5 | 93.0 | 36.6 |
| 4 years | 16.3 | 35.9 | 100.4 | 39.5 |
| 5 years | 18.3 | 40.3 | 107.2 | 42.4 |
| **Boys** | | | | |
| Birth | 3.5 | 7.7 | 54.0 | 21.3 |
| 3 months | 5.9 | 13.1 | | |
| 6 months | 7.9 | 17.4 | | |
| 9 months | 9.2 | 20.3 | | |
| 1 year | 10.2 | 22.5 | 76.3 | 30.0 |
| 2 years | 12.7 | 28.0 | 86.9 | 34.2 |
| 3 years | 14.7 | 32.4 | 94.2 | 37.1 |
| 4 years | 16.6 | 36.6 | 101.6 | 40.0 |
| 5 years | 18.5 | 40.7 | 108.3 | 42.6 |

## Height

The average length of a new baby is 50cm. By the second birthday, children are likely to have reached half their eventual adult height. Parents or carers must not become preoccupied with a child's size. If a child is happy, contented, growing and energetic there is nothing to worry about.

## Temperature

A child's normal body temperature is 36.5–37°C but this can vary depending on the time of day and the circumstances – for example, after running around the temperature will be higher than normal.

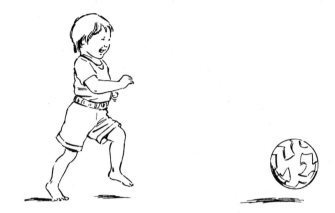

Ideally, a child's temperature should be taken using either a digital or an ear thermometer as:

- They are safe to use
- They are easy to use
- They give accurate measurements
- The figures are easy to read.

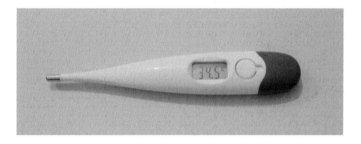

Forehead thermometers, although easy to use, are less accurate and can be difficult to read.

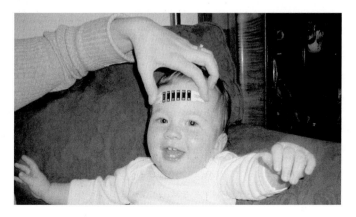

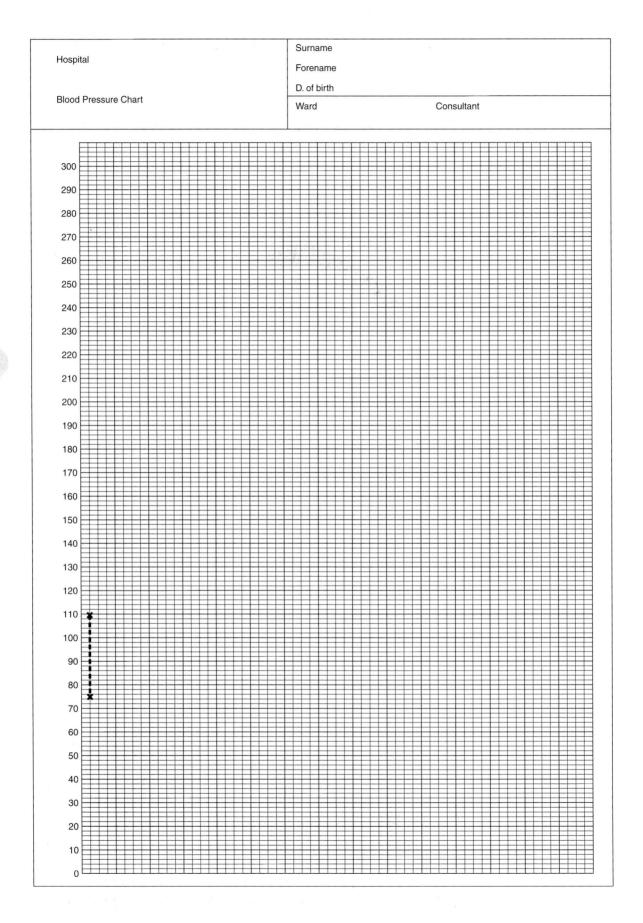

The chart on page 152 records in a graphical form the blood pressure of a service user.

## Accuracy

The student needs to be aware of potential sources of error that could occur when carrying out physiological measurements of individuals in care settings.

### Potential sources of error – reading body temperature

A glass thermometer will need to be 'shaken down' by the carer using thumb and forefinger at the opposite end to the bulb prior to use, in order for an accurate reading to be obtained. A thermometer must also be left *in situ* for the recommended length of time to ensure accuracy.

### Potential sources of error – pulse readings

The carer must use the first, second and third fingers to palpate (feel) the radial pulse; if the thumb is used for this purpose, the carer may feel his or her own pulse.

Moderate pressure should be applied in order to be able to feel the pulsation of the radial artery. Too much pressure will suppress the pulse. If too little pressure is applied, then the pulse will be difficult to locate.

### Potential sources of error – blood pressure

When using a sphygmomanometer to measure blood pressure, it is important to select a cuff of the proper width to obtain an accurate reading. If it is too narrow, the reading could be falsely high because the pressure is not evenly transmitted to the artery. This could occur, for example, when using an average-sized cuff on a person who is overweight. If a cuff is too wide, then the reading could be falsely *low,* because pressure is being directed towards a proportionately large surface area. This could occur, for example, when using an adult cuff on the thin arm of a child.

Similarly, if the cuff is too loosely wrapped around the arm, an inaccurate reading may result. Clothing that is too tight around the upper arm may also cause an inaccurate reading to be taken.

The blood pressure reading may be misleading if the measurement takes place following physical activity, or if the person is emotionally upset. The person should be at rest, assuming a comfortable sitting or lying position.

### Potential sources of error – respiratory rate

It is possible for individuals to consciously alter their own respiratory rate. It is important, therefore, to observe respiratory rate while the person is unaware, so that an accurate assessment can be made. This can be achieved by making the observation immediately after taking the pulse rate, keeping the fingers in place, so that the person is unaware that respirations are then being counted.

### Potential sources of error – lung volume

When using a spirometer, the person should not wear restrictive clothing, which may affect their breathing and, therefore, the accuracy of the result. Any medication that they are taking concerned with the respiratory tract is usually withdrawn prior to the procedure, as again a true picture of the individual's lung volume may not emerge. This must not be done without medical advice.

---

**AO6**  ## Describe physical and intellectual activities suitable for children

### Physical

Physical development is concerned with the growth and control of movement of the body. It comprises:

- Fine motor skills – manipulative skills, hand–eye co-ordination
- Gross motor skills – balance, whole-body co-ordination

Children develop these skills through a process of practice and refinement. Young children need to be given opportunities to develop these skills in both indoor and outdoor environments.

Physical exercise on large equipment helps children to develop:

- Agility
- Co-ordination
- Balance
- Confidence.

It allows them to use up excess energy and to make noise. This is particularly important for children who are learning to behave in a quiet, controlled indoor environment such as school or a nursery.

Equipment provided should give opportunities for children to exercise physically.

Physical exercise could include:

- Climbing
- Crawling
- Swimming
- Bouncing
- Sliding
- Moving around.

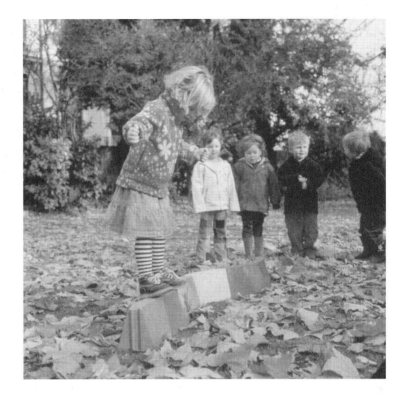

## 5

**TASK**

### Physical exercise for children

You are being interviewed for a job as a nursery nurse at a new nursery that has not yet bought any equipment. Using your knowledge and understanding of nurseries you have visited, give advice on which pieces of equipment would best encourage the physical development of the children.

### Nourishment

As has been mentioned at the beginning of this unit, it is vital that a child is well nourished, especially during the first years of life, to develop both physically and intellectually to the very best of his/her potential.

Children should eat a wide range of foods in order to gain all the necessary nutrients for growth and development.

Good eating habits should be established in early childhood. This will actively promote the development of strong bones and teeth and will prevent the child from becoming overweight or obese. This will also lay down the foundation for healthy eating throughout life.

Poor eating habits may be difficult to change during later life and could give rise to a range of diet-related problems. These include tooth decay, obesity, openness to infection and illness.

Food provides children with their energy requirements. Strenuous physical exercise such as running, skipping and hopping increases energy requirements and therefore the need for food intake.

## Creative

Children are naturally creative but must be given opportunities to explore and express their creativity.

Creativity allows children to use their ideas to make something. Creative activities can include:

- Modelling, e.g. dough, Plasticine
- Collage, e.g. fabric, pasta, pictures
- Painting
- Drawing
- Printing
- Sewing
- Making music, e.g. drums.

## Intellectual

Intellectual development is the development of thinking and learning skills.

It includes the development of the following:

- Concepts
- Creativity
- Imagination
- Problem solving
- Memory
- Concentration.

Intellectual activities such as storytelling, musical activities and puzzles all provide opportunities for the early stages of all these skills to be developed.

### Storytelling

This includes reading books suitable for the age and interests of the child. Storytelling, be it from books or made-up stories, is an important part of a child's development. Language is developed, as listening to stories enables young children to respond to the sound and rhythm of spoken language. Listening to stories extends a child's vocabulary as s/he begins to learn new words. Children have very rich imaginations and storytelling is a good way of allowing children to express a whole range of emotions.

### Musical

It is important to allow children to listen and respond to music and to provide opportunities for children to create their own music. Opportunities should be provided for children to experiment and discover how to make sounds. Children do not need musical instruments to create rhythm and sound. Everyday material can be used to improvise, such as dried peas in a tin, saucepan lids and different types of spoons.

Music is another valuable way of expressing thoughts and feelings.

### Puzzles

Puzzles represent one of the earliest examples of problem solving. Puzzles develop children's ability to sequence – this means putting stages into the correct order. In this way the brain is developed to its full potential. Puzzles also show that learning can be fun and can be a social activity where children interact with others.

## Safety

Child-care workers need to create a safe environment by identifying possible hazards and taking appropriate action to minimise the risk of accidents.

All settings have potential hazards and these need to be checked regularly.

All equipment and toys must comply with safety regulations and must be used following manufacturer's instructions.

## Comport

It is important that children from an early age conduct themselves in a manner appropriate to the activity. For example, a child riding a tricycle should sit firmly on the seat, with both feet on the pedals and both hands gripping the handlebars. Children who do not ride bikes in this manner are more likely to have an accident and injure themselves.

## Suitability

Most of us would consider playing or play to be the major recreational activity for children. Play provides physical, intellectual and social benefits. The type of play will depend upon the stage of development that the child is at. Some physical activities, such as swimming, are suitable for children of all ages. Other activities such as team games (football, hockey, netball, etc.) require physical, intellectual and social development before they are suitable. Young children may not have the physical co-ordination to catch or hit a ball, the intellectual development to understand rules, and the social development to play co-operatively in a team.

### What recreational activities are suitable for young children?

For young children, much of their recreation occurs in and around the home. Often it involves supervision and co-operation from an adult. Typical activities and the areas that they address might include:

- drawing, painting and colouring – physical and intellectual
- looking at books – intellectual
- playing with dolls – social and intellectual
- dressing up – intellectual and social
- pretend cooking – intellectual, social and physical.

## A07 Provide practical care for a child with a common childhood illness, evaluating the success of the care provided

### Providing practical care

To help you decide what practical care tasks you might carry out for a sick child you should have a long discussion with your teacher. Remember that the child's wishes and needs come first and that any thing you do must not disempower them or their parents.

### *Drawing up a plan*

Planning is an important part of carrying out any task, activity or plan. When you have selected the service user and identified the illness that they have, you will need to consider how long you have been given to carry out the plan.

### *Objective of the plan*

The plan for the sick child must include:

- Activities for intellectual stimulation (reading, board games, etc.)
- Care to meet their physical needs
- Provision of an appropriate snack.

### *Timescales*

- How long have you to carry out the activity?
- How available are any resources – the things you might need to complete the activity (facilities for intellectual activities, items for the appropriate physical care and snack)?
- Can you and the child do all you want to do in the time given?
- Do you have the individual skills to complete the activity (organisational skills, interpersonal skills, communication skills, etc.)?

How do you evaluate the effectiveness of the activity?

### Review of your activity

### *Heath and safety considerations*

When working in the health and social care services, we must always make sure that what we do does not make it hazardous for either the service user or the carer. You must, therefore, take into consideration any health and safety factors of the activities you are planning.

### How to review the activity

When you have completed the activity, you will need to review your own individual performance against the tasks that you agreed to undertake with the service user. To review the activity you will first need to look at whether you carried out the agreed activity.

You should look at:

- Whether the service user benefited from the activity
- Whether or not resources were used effectively
- Whether you dealt with any problems effectively
- Whether you maintained the health and safety of those you were working with.

### Review of your performance

To do this, you will need to look back at your original activity plan.

When reviewing what you have done, it is often a very good idea to ask the person you did the activity with, the service user, what they thought about it.

## Assessment

a) You must individually

   – Plan (the aim of the practical care, objectives, resources, timescale)

   – Set the criteria for measuring the success of the practical care

   – Carry out the practical care

   – Monitor (intellectual stimulation, the physical care, health and safety and the snack) and

   – Review the selected task.

b) You will need to consider the

   – Physical care needs of the child

   – Intellectual stimulation of the child

   – Health and safety issues

   – Snack.

c) It is very important that you consider how you can involve the child in planning the activity so as to empower them.

d) When you have carried out the chosen practical care task you must assess your own performance.

- Did you achieve the aims that you set yourself?
- Did you achieve the objectives of the practical care task?
- Did you make the best use of available resources?
- Did you meet the outcomes that you set for yourself?
- Look at your own strengths – what did you do best?
- What could you have done better?
- How did you empower the child?

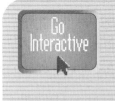

| | |
|---|---|
| BBC Newsround Online | bbc.co.uk/newsround |
| Childcare Information Service | childcare-info.co.uk |
| Childworks | childworks.co.uk |
| Cybertales | cybertales.co.uk |
| Day Care Trust | daycaretrust.org.uk |
| Grid Club | gridclub.com |
| National Day Nurseries Association | ndna.org.uk |
| Playgroup network | playgroup-network.org.uk |
| Pre-school Learning Alliance | pre-school.org.uk |
| Professional Association of Nursery Nurses | pat.org.uk |

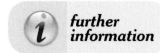

**further information**

Clarke L (2000) *Health and Social Care for Foundation GNVQ.* Nelson Thornes, Cheltenham

Clarke L (2000) *Health and Social Care for Intermediate GNVQ.* Nelson Thornes, Cheltenham

Clarke L (2002) *Health and Social Care GCSE.* NelsonThornes, Cheltenham

Marshall J and Stuart S (2001) *Child Development.* Heinemann, Oxford

Meggitt C (2001) *Baby and Child Health.* Heinemann, Oxford.

www.nhsdirect.nhs.uk – Information on child health

www.patient.co.uk/child_health.htm – Common child health problems

www.tommys.org – St Thomas' Hospital, London

www.who.int/en/ – The World Health Organisation

## Summary

- Factors affecting children's health can be lifestyle (including diet and exercise), environmental (including water quality and sewerage control), social (including health facilities and housing quality) and congenital (disorders passed from parents' genes).

- Sick children still have physical, intellectual, emotional, social and playing needs.

- There are many organisations and professionals who provide support for sick children, such as GPs, practice nurses and health visitors in a health centre.

- Common childhood infectious diseases have telltale signs and symptoms that when recognised should be acted on quickly.

- There are set procedures for performing health checks such as measuring and recording pulse, body mass index and temperature.

# 6 Health care for older service users

## To complete this unit you will need to:

- Recognise factors that affect the health of older people
- Describe the principles of caring for older people
- Describe the roles of settings and professionals who provide support for older service users when they are ill
- Identify key signs and symptoms of common illnesses affecting older service users and understand the care needs required
- Demonstrate correct health measuring, monitoring and recording techniques
- Describe physical and intellectual activities suitable for older service users
- Provide care for older service users who have common illnesses, evaluating the success of the care provided.

## Recognise factors that affect the health of older people

Today people are living longer than ever before. About 18% of the population is now over retirement age. Women tend to outlive men by about 5 years on average. The length of time a person can expect to live is known as his or her *life expectancy*.

### Introduction

Social class is a form of social stratification system for putting people into strata (layers). In the UK the Registrar-General, a government official, collects data on all births, deaths and marriages, and census data every 10 years.

Since the beginning of the 20th century, the Registrar-General has grouped people into five social classes, from a list of 20,000 jobs, as a way of classifying people. The groupings are based on the income, status, skill and educational level of each job.

Classes 1–3 are what we would usually call the middle class and Classes 4–5 might be termed working class.

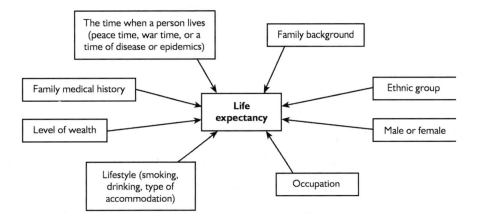

| | Class | | Examples |
|---|---|---|---|
| Middle class | 1 | Professional | Doctors, dentists, solicitors |
| | 2 | Managerial | Managers, teachers, nurses |
| | 3 | Non-manual | Clerks, typists, travel agents |
| | | Skilled manual | Electricians, hairdressers, cooks |
| Working class | 4 | Semi-skilled manual | Postmen or women, farm workers |
| | 5 | Unskilled manual | Cleaners, labourers |

*Table 6.1 The five social classes – the Registrar-General's classification*

The Registrar-General's classification has been criticised because:

- It does not take account of unemployed people
- It does not take account of people (usually women) at home looking after children or dependent relatives
- It is based on a man's occupation so that if his wife/partner has a job in a higher class, it doesn't count
- Some occupations don't fit easily into categories and there are lots of grades within individual occupations
- Individual occupations may be up- or downgraded in society before this is reflected in the scale
- People are classified by occupation – but people's lifestyle does not necessarily follow a national middle-class pattern simply because they are, say, teachers and are therefore in the middle-class bracket

● The scale doesn't necessarily reflect the power base. The people at the top don't have any more power than those at the bottom. If the refuse workers went on strike, life could become very difficult.

## The government's new social classification system

In September 1998 the government introduced a new classification system to meet the criticisms of the old system, which had so few classes. The changes were necessary because most of the population now considered itself to be middle class. The old system (which was introduced in 1921) had failed to take account of the shift towards office work and the service industries. Under the new system doctors, dentists and solicitors have slipped from the top class to the third, below the Queen and owners and managers of large companies.

*Table 6.2 The new social classification system*

| Class | Examples |
| --- | --- |
| 1 | The Queen, large company owner |
| 2 | Company executive, manager of 25 people or more |
| 3 | Doctor, lawyer, scientist, teacher, librarian, IT engineer |
| 4 | Policeman, nurse, fire-fighter, prison officer |
| 5 | Sales manager, farm manager |
| 6 | Office supervisor, civil servant, lab technician |
| 7 | Computer operator, dental nurse, secretary |
| 8 | Small business owner with under 25 employees, publican |
| 9 | Self-employed bricklayer, driving instructor |
| 10 | Factory foreman, shop supervisor, senior hairdresser |
| 11 | Craft and related workers, plumber, mechanic |
| 12–17 | + other classifications + (Un)skilled or unemployed |

## Social background

People in the higher social groups are likely to have better health care and education. Economic factors such as the amount of income we have, and how we spend it, affects how we live and is linked to social class. Obviously your income, where you live, and the job you do affects your health. The more you earn, the more money you have to spend on good-quality food and housing.

A home is a very significant factor in an individual's life. The place where we live can affect not only our physical health but also our mental health, and can even affect us socially. Poorer people are more likely to live in cheap, poor housing and in crowded conditions. Housing conditions are associated with health status in a number of ways. An obvious indicator is inadequate heating, which can give rise to hypothermia in the old and very young. Overcrowding may cause respiratory disease, and may contribute to mental health problems.

People with little or no money may not be able to pay for food or heating. Children and older people, in particular, need good, nourishing food.

## Previous working conditions

Working conditions can affect health. Think of the risk factors involved in building, working in a steel works or with heavy industrial equipment. There is no doubt that the higher up the social scale you go the better are your life chances, in terms of health, education, career opportunities and personal well-being.

## Social position

Withdrawal from the labour force does not automatically result in a reduction of social contacts with family, friends or neighbours. The more contacts the older person has before they retire the more they are likely to have after retirement.

## Lifestyle choices

Some people argue that people in the lower socioeconomic groups have worse health because of their habits, such as drinking, smoking and poor diet. People in the north, for example, have been accused of eating too much stodgy food and not enough vegetables. This sort of comment is not helpful because it blames the victim for the situation they are in rather than looking at wider issues such as poverty, which is often the root of many problems to do with lifestyle.

The comment can be described as a *deficit model*, one that makes the victim out to be deficient in some way. 'Asian mothers don't know enough about childcare and that is why the death rate of Asian babies is so high' is another example of a deficit model statement. Further questions might be asked about what makes people lower down the social scale smoke or drink more than people higher up it. What pressures are on them to resort to these things? What alternatives have they? Limited income often means limited lifestyle.

People from ethnic minority groups may find it more difficult to obtain the health care they need. Information may not be available in community languages, transport may not be available to attend hospital appointments or the demands of other children may make it impossible to sit in long queues for antenatal checks. Similar points could be made concerning white people from lower class groups.

Exercise too plays a part in health because it can improve health as well as reduce stress. An older person who has taken regular exercise throughout their life is more likely to carry on with their chosen activity once they have

*The experience of women*

Sometimes the women who immigrated to this country stayed at home caring for their families and had little contact with the indigenous population. They managed without learning much English and closely maintained their lifestyle mixing with their own people.

As women tend to outlive men, they can find themselves thrown into a strange and terrifying environment through the changes which old age inevitably brings (for example, death of a spouse, hospitalisation or ill-health).

The access to health and social services needs to be improved for all older people, but there are certain additional measures which are specially geared to the needs of ethnic elders which could be implemented with a little imagination and understanding.

Old age is often viewed in a negative way – as a stage of life that just brings problems, such as the need for residential accommodation or health and social care. But people do not change simply because they have reached old age. Many remain independent for most, if not all, of their lives.

Old age can be divided into two stages:

- Early old age (up to 75 years)
- Late old age (beyond 75 years).

## The needs of older people

We build up relationships with service users by showing them that we have up-to-date knowledge about the services that are available and how these services can help them.

Before you can give any advice, however, you need to find out what a service user's needs are. How do you do this? First you have to carry out an assessment of the service user's situation.

We also build relationships with service users by showing them that we have up-to-date knowledge about the services that are available and how these services can help them. Before you can give any advice, however, you need to find out what a service user's needs are. How do you do this? First you have to carry out an assessment of the service user's situation – his or her abilities, expectations and aspirations. You do this by looking at the service user's needs under the following headings:

- Physical needs
- Emotional needs
- Intellectual needs
- Social and cultural needs.

## How are a service user's needs assessed?

### *Maslow's theory of human needs*

This theory is a useful starting point. Maslow suggests that human needs are arranged in a series of five levels, as shown in Figure 6.2. The needs at level 1, such as shelter, food and water, are the basic, essential requirements for any individual to live. The more complex needs shown from the middle of the pyramid upwards are only considered when the basic needs have been taken care of. For example, a homeless, hungry person needs shelter and food before they might worry about their social needs.

*Maslow's hierarchy of needs*

**5 Self actualisation:**
Fulfilment, use of creative talents

**4 Esteem needs:**
Self-respect, need to feel competent and respected

**3 Social/love needs:**
Need to belong, to associate and participate in groups

**2 Safety needs:**
Freedom from fear, deprivation, danger or threat

**1 Basic physical needs:**
Shelter, food, water, other basics for survival

- **Level 1: Basic physical needs** – These include the need to satisfy hunger and thirst, the need for oxygen and the need to keep warm or cool. These also include the need for sleep, sensory pleasures, maternal behaviour and sexual desire. If people are denied any of these needs, they may spend long periods of time looking for them. For example, if water or food is not readily available, most people's energies will be spent trying to obtain a supply.

- **Level 2: Safety needs** – Once basic physical needs have been met, a person's next concern is usually for safety and security, freedom from pain and from threat of physical attack, and protection from danger.

- **Level 3: Love and social needs** – These include affection, a sense of belonging, the need for social activities, friendships, and the giving and receiving of love.

- **Level 4: Self-esteem needs** – These include the need to have self-respect and to have the esteem of others. Self-respect involves the desire to have confidence, strength, independence, freedom and achievement. The esteem of others involves having prestige, status, recognition, attention, reputation and appreciation from other people.

- **Level 5: Self actualisation/self-fulfilment needs** – This is the development and realisation of your full potential. All the other needs in the pyramid have to be achieved before you can reach this stage.

### Activities of daily living

Another way to assess a service user's needs is by using the 'activities of daily living' model. The assessor looks at the service user's situation in relation to the everyday activities that people need to carry out. The activities include:

- **Safe environment** – freedom from pain, comfort
- **Body functions** – breathing comfortably, passing urine and faeces regularly, maintaining body temperature, etc.
- **Nutrition** – a healthy diet, ability to eat, adequate and suitable fluids
- **Personal cleaning and dressing** – mouth, teeth, eyes, ears, skin, suitable clothing, ability to dress and undress
- **Mobility** – can the service user get out of bed or exercise?
- **Sleep** – sleep pattern, does the service user wake during the night or sleep during the day?
- **Sexuality** – is the service user able to express their feelings? Do they have the ability to enter into meaningful sexual relationships?
- **Religion** – are the cultural needs of service user being met? Do they have the freedom to worship as they wish?
- **Communication** – is the service user able to communicate verbally, express emotions, use smell, touch?

## How are people's needs met?

### Physical needs

These may be met by:

- The provision of appropriate food and drink – for example, babies and people who are ill (such as someone suffering from diabetes) need different diets from a healthy adult
- Attending to personal hygiene – this is essential to prevent infection and spread of disease.

### Intellectual and emotional needs

These may be more difficult to meet. It is important to:

- Treat people as individuals

- Respect people's individuality and opinions
- Allow people to be as independent as possible.

For example, in a residential home for elderly people these needs may be met by allowing residents to:

- Be independent
- Choose their own meals
- Make decisions about their own meal times, bed times, visiting times
- Participate in social and educational activities in the establishment and outside of it.

Emotional needs are not separate from physical needs. People often feel better after a bath or a visit to the hairdresser. If they feel clean, they feel more secure when interacting with others. For example, someone who smells of urine will not feel emotionally secure when talking to relatives or friends. By meeting their physical need, their emotional need may also be met.

### Social and cultural needs

These are an important aspect of a person's life. Social needs can be met by:

- Encouraging people to socialise
- Encouraging people to keep in touch with relatives and friends
- Arranging for volunteers to visit them in their own homes if they are housebound.

Cultural needs are recognised when people are allowed to practise their cultural rituals and traditions. They can be met by recognising that people:

- Need to practise their religion
- Have cultural food preferences
- Relate to individuals in their family according to their cultural practices.

### Safety needs

As a person ages, the senses can deteriorate, leaving them more vulnerable to accidents both inside and outside the home. Falls are

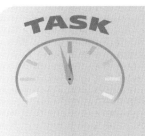

### TASK

### Home safety for older people

Home safety is very high-profile with Age Concern, who run a safety check programme called A.P.P.L.E.S.

Contact this voluntary organisation and find out about the A.P.P.L.E.S. programme in your area.

common among the over-75 age group. However, certain precautions can be taken to prevent falls:

- Ensure all areas are well lit
- Try to have all necessary living facilities on one floor, i.e. as in a flat
- If living in a two-storey house, have a downstairs and upstairs toilet so that there is no unnecessary climbing of stairs
- Install handrails, bath rails and stair lift if necessary.

Other problems related to failing senses are:

- **Hearing loss**
  - Cannot hear cars until too close
  - Cannot hear shouted warnings
- **Failing sight**
  - Cannot see cars until very close
  - Can trip over something that they did not see
- **Failing sense of smell**
  - Cannot smell gas
  - Cannot smell burning
- **Failing sense of touch**
  - Hot water bottle too hot – burns legs or feet
  - Sits too near fire and burns legs
  - Feels cold too late and has already developed hypothermia
- **Loss of memory**
  - Forgets to turn off oven or burner when cooking
  - Forgets to turn off iron or kettle
  - Forgets to turn off tap
  - Forgets whether or not they have already taken medication.

**Case Study**

Mrs. Telford is 84 years old. She lives in her own home and feels that she can manage to look after herself and run the house. Recently she was nearly knocked down by a double-decker bus. A week later she slipped on the stairs at home but fortunately only suffered severe bruising. A neighbour saved her kitchen from burning down after she left a frying pan of bacon and sausages on the gas burner and they caught fire.

*Read through the scenario carefully. Do you think Mrs. Telford's senses are failing. If so, which ones?*

To try to prevent accidents due to failing senses:

- Encourage older people to cross the road at a pelican or zebra crossing
- Have smoke alarms fitted
- Put medication into daily-dose boxes
- Instead of a hot water bottle, have an electric blanket that switches off when the correct temperature is reached
- Have a fire guard around the fire
- Set the central heating thermostat at 20°C to maintain room temperature.

Can you think of any more?

### Intellectual stimulation

Many older people maintain a healthy, independent lifestyle. They organise their lives to meet their recreational needs. It is not this group that we will consider in this section. For some older people, specific recreational support is needed. Those who live alone may need support in maintaining social activities. Others may have very little mobility and need assistance in physical activity. It may also be necessary to provide intellectual stimulation.

Facilities available that provide recreation specifically for older people include day centres and residential homes. Some leisure centres also run specific sessions to support the recreation needs of older people.

Day centres and residential homes provide a variety of activities. For example, they provide a place where people meet socially, offering opportunities for conversation and other forms of social recreation. They also provide intellectual recreation in a variety of ways:

- They often offer the opportunity to play games, both group games, such as bingo, and individual challenges, such as chess and draughts.
- For some people, intellectual stimulation has to be organised on a one-to-one basis by the care workers. Conversation with care workers, involving remembering things that have happened in the past, is important. Using photographs and things from the past to stimulate memories also enables people to think about the present.
- Intellectual recreation can also include activities related to occupational therapy. Intellectual activity may come from concentrating on painting, sewing or knitting. It may come from practising a skill like cooking. All of these also provide a degree of physical activity. They do not provide exercise like swimming, but they require fine movements and help maintain hand and finger mobility.

### Social contact

Social relationships are very important to an older person, as they make them feel alive and in touch with the world around them. Social contact helps their intellectual development and keeps their minds active. If an older person lives alone they can easily feel cut off from other people. A conversation stimulates them and makes them feel good about themselves and their environment.

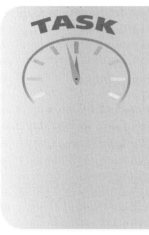

## TASK

### The social and intellectual needs of older people

In your community, find out about the clubs, groups and other opportunities available to the elderly for recreation which will promote social contact and intellectual stimulation.

Make a list, e.g.:

- Bingo.

Visit a care home for the elderly near you. Find out about the opportunities for social contact and intellectual stimulation available to the residents.

 **AO3** **Describe the roles of settings and professionals who provide support for older service users when they are ill**

### Health centres

The health centre would be the first place for an older person to visit. The health centre staff are the primary care team, meaning that they look after health care in the community. The team can consist of one or several of the following:

- GP
- Practice nurse
- Community nurse
- Health visitor
- Midwife.

There are several other health professionals that the practice will have access to:

- Chiropodist
- Physiotherapist
- Occupational therapist
- Speech therapist
- Counsellor
- Social worker.

The main professionals from the above lists who deal with the older person are as follows.

### The GP

The GP will:

- Diagnose and give treatment for illness

- Refer patients to secondary health care (e.g. a hospital) if necessary
- Refer patients to other team members if necessary.

### The practice nurse

Older people might have injections given to them or blood samples, blood pressure and urine samples taken by the practice nurse.

### The community nurse

The job of the community nurse (formerly the district nurse) is to offer nursing care to patients in their own homes. A high proportion of the community nurse's work tends to be with older patients who wish to stay in their own homes as long as they can. The community nurse will monitor patients as part of the visit.

The community nurse might be expected to:

- Give injections
- Change dressings
- Monitor blood pressure
- Take blood samples
- Give a bed bath
- Arrange for GP to visit.

### The health visitor

The older person will be offered advice by the health visitor on how to keep fit and healthy and how to prevent illness. Health visitors play a large part in the community care of older people.

### The chiropodist

The chiropodist will care for the older service user's feet, dealing with such complaints as corns, ingrowing toenails and hammer toes. The majority of people who receive this service are 65 or over.

### The social worker

A social worker will assess the older person's and his/her carer's individual needs and organise services with other professionals to meet these.

### The physiotherapist

Physiotherapists have an important role in improving the mobility of patients, using supportive and manipulative exercises to develop muscles for movement. Physiotherapists improve the health and function of service users through simple corrective exercises. They help older people after they have had a stroke.

### The speech therapist

Speech therapists help people with speech disorders. Although most of their work is with children, they will help older people recovering from strokes.

## Secondary health care

Secondary health care describes hospital services, as they are usually the second part of treatment after patients have first been to their doctor. People can be admitted for treatment or attend the hospital as outpatients at a clinic. An outpatient comes to the hospital for one or more of the following:

- Health screening, such as electrocardiography (ECG), X-ray, endoscopy, etc.
- To see a consultant, who is a doctor who specialises in specific types of complaint or disease
- Any therapy, such as physiotherapy, occupational or speech therapy
- Ongoing treatment such as radiotherapy or chemotherapy.

### The geriatrician

A geriatrician is a doctor who specialises in treating older people and the diseases that usually occur in old age, for example Alzheimer's disease.

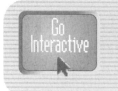

**Find out about careers in the National Health Service using this website:**

- nhscareers.nhs.uk

### Clinics

As already mentioned, the older person can attend various clinics as an outpatient. Women up to the age of 70 can attend breast cancer screening clinics.

## Professional support workers

Earlier in this unit the roles and responsibilities of many of the people involved in supporting and providing physical assistance to older people were discussed. We looked at the support that professional workers such as the physiotherapist, the social worker, the GP and nurses can provide. The figure on page 177 shows all the services that could be involved in delivering physical assistance and emotional support to an older person with a disability.

*Professional support workers*

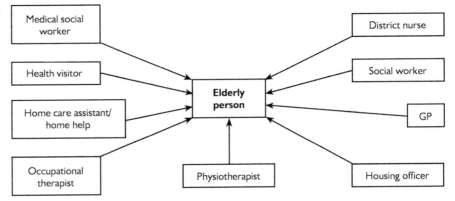

As you can see from this diagram, there are many people involved, providing services and assistance. All these people must work together to provide the best service possible. It is also important that they co-operate very closely with relatives and friends of the service user.

However, most important of all is that everyone, professional workers and carers, must take into account, and act upon, the wishes of the service user. What the service user wants is the most important thing, not what is available to offer them or what we as carers might think is the best thing for them. It is the older person who must have the final say in what services and support they want. So that the service user can make informed decisions, the carer should:

- Explain what process they are involved in
- Let the service user put forward their own views
- Agree with the service user what services they would wish
- Talk through with the service user how the services can be delivered
- Involve the service user fully in reviewing the situation as appropriate.

The figure on page 178 shows the different organisations that may be involved in offering support.

## Support groups to help older people with dependent needs

The voluntary organisations play an important role in the provision of care for elderly, dependent people. They can be very flexible in the services they provide and how they provide them. They are not bound by the rules and regulations that may hinder statutory services.

Voluntary organisations and self-help groups can be of great help to elderly people, particularly those who are housebound. They can:

- Provide information about services available and help people get appropriate support
- Provide information about assistive equipment

- Pain killers
- Anti-inflammatory drugs
- Regular exercise.

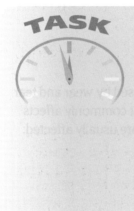

## Understanding what it is like to have arthritis

Wearing a thick, man's sock over each hand, try to carry out the following tasks:

- Button a shirt or blouse
- Tie shoe laces
- Eat a yoghurt with a small spoon
- Write your name.

How difficult did you find each task?

## Rheumatism

This is the common name for pain and stiffness in muscles and joints. Rheumatism can be brought on by a number of different factors, for example cold weather, stress or poor posture. Older people tend to suffer from rheumatism, as muscle and joint aches and pains increase with age.

### Treatment

The following may help:

- Pain killers
- Exercise
- Keeping weight down
- Keeping affected areas warm.

## Osteoporosis

Our reduced ability to absorb calcium in middle and old age means that some may be lost from the skeleton and not replaced. This makes the bones more likely to wear or break. It also means that breaks take longer to heal. This condition is called osteoporosis. Women, during and after the menopause, are at most risk. During the menopause the ovaries stop producing hormones as well as stopping egg production. This change in the body's hormone balance means that calcium loss increases.

### Symptoms

- Severe headache
- Fracture of bones.

*Professional support workers*

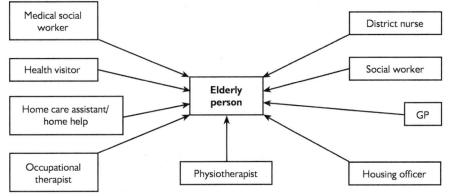

As you can see from this diagram, there are many people involved, providing services and assistance. All these people must work together to provide the best service possible. It is also important that they co-operate very closely with relatives and friends of the service user.

However, most important of all is that everyone, professional workers and carers, must take into account, and act upon, the wishes of the service user. What the service user wants is the most important thing, not what is available to offer them or what we as carers might think is the best thing for them. It is the older person who must have the final say in what services and support they want. So that the service user can make informed decisions, the carer should:

- Explain what process they are involved in
- Let the service user put forward their own views
- Agree with the service user what services they would wish
- Talk through with the service user how the services can be delivered
- Involve the service user fully in reviewing the situation as appropriate.

The figure on page 178 shows the different organisations that may be involved in offering support.

## Support groups to help older people with dependent needs

The voluntary organisations play an important role in the provision of care for elderly, dependent people. They can be very flexible in the services they provide and how they provide them. They are not bound by the rules and regulations that may hinder statutory services.

Voluntary organisations and self-help groups can be of great help to elderly people, particularly those who are housebound. They can:

- Provide information about services available and help people get appropriate support
- Provide information about assistive equipment

*Organisations offering support and physical assistance to elderly, dependent service users*

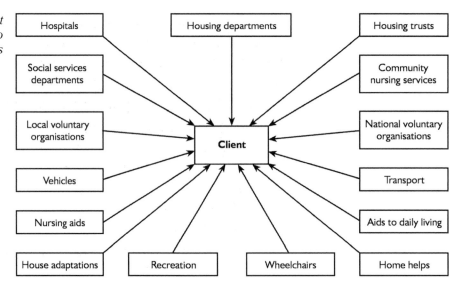

- Visit and provide support – Age Concern, for example, provides a wide range of services for older people:

  - Visiting service for older people, offering companionship

  - Good neighbour scheme, provision of visiting, shopping, gardening and other household tasks

  - Holidays

  - Telephone link – volunteers contact the housebound older person at pre-arranged time each day to check they are OK and also to offer support

  - Day centres

  - Coffee shops and luncheon clubs

  - Free transport.

## Who gives care?

Other groups, such as the Association of Stroke Clubs, provide self-help and information to members. Cross-roads is a voluntary scheme providing a support system for people in their own homes by offering temporary or regular care relief. This provides support and a rest for the carer by allowing the volunteer to attend to the personal needs of the service user. Six million people are involved in providing voluntary services in the UK. The day-to-day work that the volunteers do is varied. They offer an informal system of caring that bridges the gap between the older service user and the statutory services.

### Community and Social Services

Social Services Departments were set up by local authorities in the late 1960s to provide community-based services for people in their own homes.

The service is available to everyone, but is particularly concerned with families. The Social Services Committee of every local authority (council) oversees the four main responsibilities of its Social Services Department:

- To provide childcare as specified in the various Children's Acts and Adoption Acts, including the 1989 Children Act

- To provide and regulate residential accommodation for older people and people with disabilities, as specified in the 1948 National Assistance Act and the 1984 Registered Homes Act

- To provide welfare services for older people, people with disabilities and people who are chronically (long-term) ill and to act as set out in the various Mental Health Acts

- To refer service users to other organisations, such as voluntary organisations, for services.

*Jobs in community services involved with the elderly*

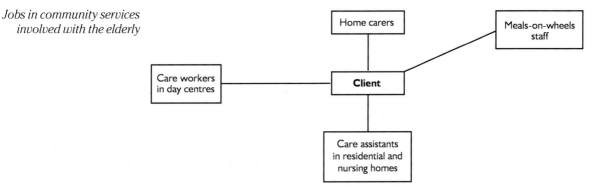

### Home care staff

A number of staff provide everyday emotional, social and practical support to service users living in their own homes. By law, local authorities must provide home care assistants (formerly called home helps). They carry out such tasks as:

- Simple cleaning
- Lighting fires
- Shopping
- Cooking
- Basic personal tasks.

Most of their work is concerned with supporting elderly people but they do also work with people with physical disabilities and families with young children.

### Meals-on-wheels

This service is becoming increasingly important as more and more dependent older people choose to carry on living in their own homes. About 33 million meals are provided every year to people in their own homes in England. This service is provided by the local authority in many areas but it is still also offered by voluntary agencies such as the Women's Royal Voluntary Service (WRVS) or, in rural areas, the Women's Institute (WI).

### The care assistant

The job of a basic-grade care assistant looking after elderly people, either in a day centre or in residential care, is the first rung on the ladder of a career in health and social care.

Older people can seek help, advice and support from any of the professionals mentioned in this unit. Obviously medical staff, such as GPs and nurses, are qualified to give advice on medication and screening.

## Hospitalisation of older people

### Emotional reaction

Even though older people realise that going in to hospital will benefit them in the long term, they will be worried. Fear about leaving their home, family and pets, as well as about the treatment, will make them feel vulnerable. A good GP/health professional will help them to feel that they have some control over what happens to them in hospital, by establishing a good relationship with them. To make a stay in hospital less stressful, patients should be:

- Involved in their own treatment by having everything about their illness explained to them so they feel informed
- Allowed and encouraged to make choices for themselves
- Respected regarding their wishes and opinions
- Seen as an individual and not as an 'illness' (e.g. 'a diabetic') or an 'old person'.

Health and social care services should be able to respond flexibly and sensitively to the needs of the service user. This allows the service user to feel independent and prevents their condition from getting worse.

### Preparing for visits/pre-admission activities

The members of the primary care team can prepare the older person for their stay in hospital – answering any questions about the treatment that they have. Pre-admission procedures will also be explained by the team. The hospital will send leaflets and a letter with specific instructions – for example, if the person is having a local anaesthetic they may asked to have nothing to eat after 6 pm the evening before admission.

### The stay in hospital

It is important for all older people to become familiar with the layout of the hospital ward. This will allow them autonomy and enable the older person to feel in control and empowered.

The older person should be introduced to the ward staff and what is going to happen to them (treatment, etc.) explained so that they feel safe and will not be frightened by the unexpected or unfamiliar.

The staff should answer all questions clearly and as honestly as possible.

### Convalescence

This is the recovery period following an illness or surgical operation. During convalescence the patient will regain strength before returning to normal activities. Before sending the older person home after their treatment, the hospital social worker will ensure that there is someone at home to look after them. The community nurse will visit to change dressings and to check on progress. During this period the convalescent will require some bed rest, perhaps in the form of an afternoon nap, depending on the severity of the operation/treatment. Plenty of light, nutritious food will be necessary in order to regain lost strength. It is good for convalescents to have visitors, as it will make them feel better.

**Case Study**

Mr. Anderson is 69 years old and lives with his wife. He has been a builder all his working life. He has developed a hernia, which has been causing him a lot of pain over the past year. He has now been given a date for his operation. It will be the first time in his life that he has been in hospital, as he has always been healthy. He is worried, so his wife has persuaded him to talk to the practice nurse about his concerns.

*What does Mrs. Anderson need to do to help her husband convalesce when he returns home?*

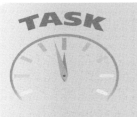

**TASK**

### Case study – Mr Anderson

In pairs, talk about the issues you feel are connected with Mr. Anderson's hospitalisation.

Using role play, demonstrate how the practice nurse could reassure Mr. Anderson, so that he felt confident about going in to hospital.

6

**Identify key signs and symptoms of common illnesses affecting older service users and understand the care needs required**

## Hyperthermia

Hyperthermia is when the body temperature is dangerously above the normal body heat of 36.5–37.2°C. A high temperature is the result of bacteria invading the body. It is a common symptom of illness. See Unit 5 for a more detailed explanation.

### Symptoms

- Shivering
- Sweating
- Flushed face
- Hot skin
- Thirst.

### Treatment

- Give older person aspirin or paracetamol to bring down their temperature
- Give plenty of cool drinks to replace fluid lost through sweating
- Remove quilts and cover with cotton sheet
- Sponge forehead with tepid water.

## Hypothermia

Hypothermia is when the body temperature falls below 35°C. It is usually caused by spending time in a cold place without being wrapped up well enough. The condition is very serious, and can cause death in older people.

### Symptoms

- Body temperature below 35°C
- Slow pulse
- Pale skin
- Slow movements
- Drowsiness
- Unconsciousness in severe cases.

### Treatment

- Hypothermia is a medical emergency and an ambulance must be called
- If the person is conscious, cover them with blankets or a quilt
- Offer warm drinks
- The room should be heated gradually to 25°C.
- If the person is unconscious, place them in the recovery position.

## Arthritis

There are two main types of arthritis:

- Osteoarthritis
- Rheumatoid arthritis.

### Osteoarthritis

This is the most common type of arthritis and is caused by wear and tear on the joints. It usually starts in middle age and most commonly affects older people. The larger and most often used joints are usually affected:

- Knees
- Hands
- Hips
- Ankles
- Feet.

Symptoms

- Pain when using affected joints
- Swelling and restriction of joint movement.

Treatment

There is no cure, but the following may help to relieve the symptoms:

- Hip replacement
- Anti-inflammatory drugs
- Pain killers
- Physiotherapy
- Exercises
- Walking
- Keeping weight down.

### Rheumatoid arthritis

This is the most severe type of arthritis. It is sometimes found in quite young people and usually affects the smaller joints:

- Fingers
- Hands
- Shoulders
- Elbows
- Wrists.

More women than men suffer from rheumatoid arthritis, and even children can have it. However, there are also many older people who suffer from it.

Symptoms

- Joints swell and are painful, hot and stiff
- Joints become deformed.

Treatment

Again there is no cure, but the following may help:

- Physiotherapy
- Weight loss

- Pain killers
- Anti-inflammatory drugs
- Regular exercise.

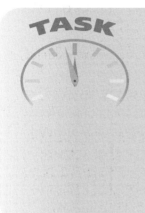

**TASK**

## Understanding what it is like to have arthritis

Wearing a thick, man's sock over each hand, try to carry out the following tasks:

- Button a shirt or blouse
- Tie shoe laces
- Eat a yoghurt with a small spoon
- Write your name.

How difficult did you find each task?

## Rheumatism

This is the common name for pain and stiffness in muscles and joints. Rheumatism can be brought on by a number of different factors, for example cold weather, stress or poor posture. Older people tend to suffer from rheumatism, as muscle and joint aches and pains increase with age.

### Treatment

The following may help:

- Pain killers
- Exercise
- Keeping weight down
- Keeping affected areas warm.

## Osteoporosis

Our reduced ability to absorb calcium in middle and old age means that some may be lost from the skeleton and not replaced. This makes the bones more likely to wear or break. It also means that breaks take longer to heal. This condition is called osteoporosis. Women, during and after the menopause, are at most risk. During the menopause the ovaries stop producing hormones as well as stopping egg production. This change in the body's hormone balance means that calcium loss increases.

### Symptoms

- Severe headache
- Fracture of bones.

### Treatment

Osteoporosis cannot be cured and the best treatment is prevention by:

- Making sure a diet rich in calcium and vitamin D is eaten earlier in life
- Exercising regularly
- Hormone replacement therapy (HRT) (although this is controversial)
- Not smoking.

**Case Study**

Ms Watson is a single career woman in her mid fifties. She is at the top of her profession, which is very stressful. Eating is not high on her list of priorities. She tends to snatch snacks when she can. She starts each day with two cups of black coffee and maintains this caffeine intake throughout the day, supplemented with cigarettes. On average she smokes about 35 cigarettes a day, and this can even be 50 when she is feeling stressed. Because of her long working hours, Ms Watson does not have time for physical exercise.

Six months ago Ms Watson stumbled off the escalator at work in her high heels, fell and fractured her left wrist. This fracture has taken a long time to heal. Recently, Ms Watson has started to suffer from severe, persistent backache.

*Consider this scenario very carefully and list the reasons why Ms Watson could be a candidate for osteoporosis.*

*How can Ms Watson prevent osteoporosis from developing?*

## High blood pressure

This is when the pressure of the blood pumping around the body is higher than normal. It can lead to a stroke if it goes unchecked.

### Symptoms

- Sometimes none
- Headaches
- Giddiness
- Shortage of breath
- Chest pains.

### Treatment

- Give up smoking
- Try to lose weight
- Take exercise
- Restrict amount of salt consumed
- Cut down on intake of foods rich in animal fats.

In case of very high blood pressure, known as *hypertension*, the older person may have to take prescribed medication.

## Respiratory system conditions

### Common cold

This is a viral infection, which causes inflammation of the mucous membranes lining the nose and throat.

Symptoms

- Sneezing
- Running nose
- Stuffy nose
- Headache
- Sore throat.

Treatment

There is no immediate cure, but older patients should keep warm.

- Drink plenty of fluids
- Warm drinks, particularly of honey, lemon juice and hot water, help to relieve sore throats
- Pain killers may relieve aches and pains.

### Influenza

Influenza is a viral infection of the respiratory tract.

Symptoms

- Headache
- Fever/chills
- Tiredness and fatigue
- Muscular aches
- Sore throat
- Runny nose
- Loss of appetite.

Treatment

- Bed rest in a warm, well-ventilated room
- Lots of warm drinks
- Pain killers to relieve aches and pains.

If secondary infection develops, particularly in older people who have a lung or heart disease, then this could lead to pneumonia, which is life-threatening. Therefore the older patient needs to be carefully monitored to ensure that symptoms are clearing up.

It is recommended that older people (over 60) have the influenza vaccine injection each autumn.

## Bronchitis

Bronchitis is an inflammation of the lining of the air tubes of the lungs, the bronchi. Acute bronchitis usually follows a cold, a sore throat or influenza, most often in winter. It is very common as a winter flare-up in people with chronic bronchitis. It may also be brought on by breathing a polluted atmosphere or by smoking.

In most cases the condition settles within a week or two, but there is always the risk, especially in cigarette smokers, that the condition may progress to chronic bronchitis with inevitable winter flare-ups.

Chronic bronchitis is one of the forms of chronic obstructive lung (pulmonary) disease (COPD). In the early stages chronic bronchitis may be a comparatively mild disease. But, with time and continued abuse, it is likely to progress to chronic obstructive airway disease (COAD), in which large numbers of the tiny lung air sacs break down to form a smaller number of larger air spaces. The total surface area now available for transferring oxygen to the blood is much less, so the person becomes short of oxygen. In addition, the smaller bronchial tubes become inflamed, narrowed and partially blocked by mucus. The result is increased breathlessness.

## Asthma

Many adults suffer from asthma. It is more common in men than in women. Asthma also occurs later in life in individuals who suffer from chronic bronchitis.

### Symptoms

- Coughing
- Wheezing
- Difficulty in breathing out
- Tight feeling in chest
- Raised pulse.

### Treatment

- If the person is lying down, sit them up in a comfortable position. In many cases the person themselves will know what position is most comfortable. Sometimes a person suffering cannot bear to be touched and may want all their clothes loosened. Lean them slightly forward. In this position it is easier to use the chest muscles for breathing. Make sure there is plenty of fresh air available by opening a window.
- If this is a first attack, a doctor or ambulance should be called.
- Give plenty of reassurance until the doctor or ambulance arrives. The person will be very frightened when they have difficulty breathing.
- If the person knows that they suffer from asthma, they probably have an inhaler. Find out where their inhaler is. Get it and help them to use it.

## Signs, symptoms and care for bowel conditions

### Gastroenteritis

This is inflammation of the stomach and intestines, and can be caused by bacteria or a virus.

Symptoms

- Appetite loss
- Nausea
- Vomiting
- Stomach pains or cramps
- Diarrhoea.

Treatment

- Bed rest
- Plenty of fluids – small amounts sipped regularly
- No solids until symptoms disappear.

If severe, this condition may have to be treated in hospital, where the patient will be given fluids by an intravenous drip. Severe symptoms, such as dehydration, shock and collapse, are most likely in the very young and in older people. The important issue here is to ensure that the older person is replacing lost fluids. If worried, call for the doctor.

### Diverticular disease

This is a bowel disease in which *diverticula* (small protruding sacs) form in the wall of the intestine. They become inflamed when faecal material gathers in them.

Symptoms

- Constipation
- Diarrhoea
- Bleeding from rectum/anus
- Abdominal pain.

Treatment

- High fibre diet
- Antibiotics.

### Irritable bowel syndrome

Irritable bowel syndrome is a bowel disease that is twice as common in women as it is in men. It usually begins in early or middle adulthood and basically it is an irritation of the large intestine.

Symptoms

- Excessive wind
- Cramp-like pains in abdomen

- Constipation
- Diarrhoea.

Treatment
- High fibre diet
- Reduction of stressful situations (if possible)
- The doctor can prescribe drugs to relieve muscular spasms.

Although treatment can help symptoms, there is no cure. The condition is not life-threatening.

### Ulcerative colitis

This is a bowel disease causing chronic inflammation of the large bowel.

Symptoms
- Pain
- Bloody diarrhoea.

Treatment
- Fruit-free diet
- Steroids to reduce inflammation.

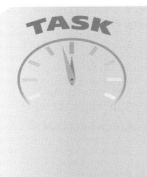

## TASK

### Fibre goes a long way to prevent bowel disease

Compare the fibre content, per 100 grams, listed on the back of cereal packets:

- Cornflakes
- Shredded Wheat
- Coco Pops
- Porridge Oats
- Muesli
- Bran Buds.

Which has the highest fibre content?

## AO5 — Demonstrate correct health measuring, monitoring and recording techniques

### Temperature

In most people the body temperature varies between 36.5°C and 37.2°C. It is affected by factors such as sleep, exercise, eating and drinking, and time of day. The usual way of taking an older person's temperature is either under the tongue or in the armpit. This can be done with a traditional clinical thermometer or an electronic thermometer. The principles of taking an oral temperature, however, remain the same:

1. The equipment (thermometer, wipes, chart, pen) should be prepared
2. The patient/service user should receive an explanation about the procedure
3. The nurse/carer should wash his/her hands
4. The thermometer should be cleaned.

## Pulse

Each time the heart beats to pump blood, a wave passes along the walls of the arteries. This wave is the pulse and it can be felt at any point in the body where a large artery crosses a bone just beneath the skin. The pulse is usually counted at the radial artery in the wrist or the carotid artery in the neck. To take a pulse, the fingertips (but not the thumb tips) are placed over the site where the pulse is being taken. The beats are counted for a full minute and then recorded. Normally the rhythm is regular and the volume is sufficient to make the pulse easily felt. The three main observations, which are made on the pulse, are rate, rhythm and strength.

The average adult pulse rate varies between 60 and 80 beats per minute, while a young baby has a heart rate of about 140 beats per minute. An increased pulse rate may indicate recent exercise, emotion, infection, blood or fluid loss, shock and heart disease.

## Peak flow/lung volume

The measurement of air taken into and expelled from the lungs is called *spirometry*. Changes in lung volumes provide the best measurement of obstruction to air flow in the respiratory passages.

A spirometer consists of a hollow drum floating over a chamber of water and counterbalanced by weights, so that it can move freely up and down.

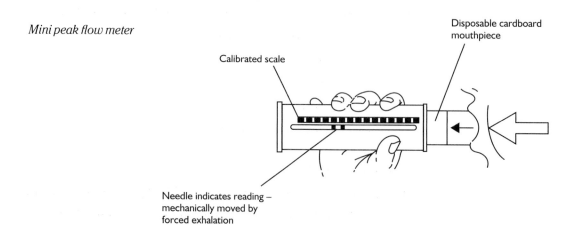

*Mini peak flow meter*

Disposable cardboard mouthpiece

Calibrated scale

Needle indicates reading – mechanically moved by forced exhalation

Inside the drum is a mixture of gases, usually oxygen and air. Leading from the hollow space in the drum to the outside is a tube that has a mouthpiece through which the patient breathes. As s/he inhales and exhales through the tube, the drum rises and falls, causing a needle to move on a nearby rotating chart. The tracing recorded is called a *spirogram*.

Various measurements are made of lung capacity. *Vital capacity* refers to the volume of air breathed out after a person has breathed in as fully as possible. The normal capacity is approximately 2500–3000 millilitres (ml). It is higher in males than females. Forced vital capacity measurements are taken in the form of *peak flow measurement*.

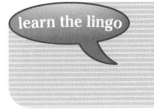

**Forced vital capacity** is the total amount of air someone can breath out by trying as hard as possible to empty the lungs. **Peak flow** is the most air per second that someone can blow out. This is what is measured by a peak flow meter.

Vital capacity is reduced in obstructive lung diseases, such as bronchitis (inflammation of the bronchi, the large air passages in the lungs). A person suffering from asthma would also have a reduced vital capacity, due to difficulty in breathing because of muscular spasm of the bronchi.

## Height and weight

### Body mass index

We are all familiar with our own body size and shape. Looking around, we can see there is an immense variation in others' sizes and shapes. We are all individuals. If, however, a person is underweight, this can be an indicator of their physical health. The body mass index is often used to measure this aspect of health. Body mass index (BMI) can be calculated by dividing a person's weight (in kilograms) by the square of their height (in metres). This can then be used as a guide to five BMI groups:

- Underweight: BMI 19.9 and below
- Normal: BMI 20–24.9
- Overweight: BMI 25–29.9
- Obese: BMI 30–39.9
- Severely obese: BMI 40 and above.

### Average or normal

It is important to remember that it is possible to be different from the average in height, weight, etc. but still be within normal limits.

**6**

**Case Study**

Mrs Patel is 58 years old. She is 1.70m (5ft 7in) tall, and weighs 90kg (14 stone). She loves eating fast food and also eats snacks between meals. She likes several glasses of wine in the evening, and enjoys eating family-sized bags of crisps. She takes no physical exercise.

*Using national standards (BMI and the height/weight chart) measure and plot Mrs Patel's weight. Does she need to lose weight?*

*What is Mrs. Patel's weight considered to be by national standards?*

The following figure shows the heights and weights of adults. To find out whether you need to lose or gain weight, draw a line up from your weight and across from your height. Mark a cross where the two lines meet.

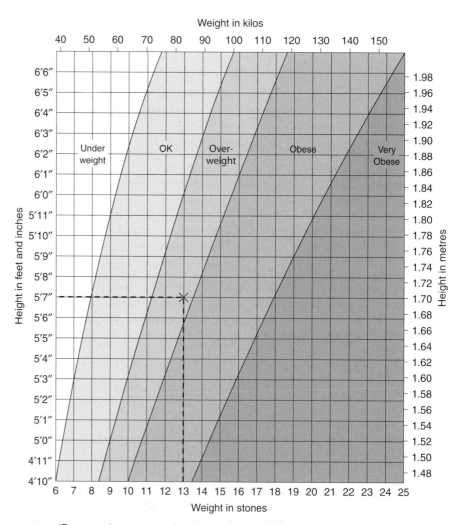

(For example, a person who is 5'7" tall and weighs 13 stones is overweight)

**AO6** **Describe physical and intellectual activities suitable for older service users**

See AO2 for advice on physical and intellectual needs.

## Physical activities

### Exercise

Being older is no barrier to taking part in and enjoying regular exercise. The benefits can be enormous and can have a very positive impact on the outlook upon life. Exercise naturally relaxes both the mind and the body, as it induces a sense of well-being. Exercise also lowers stress levels, which lowers blood pressure and helps maintain a healthy heart and lungs. It benefits the muscles and joints and helps balance and co-ordination.

It is important to consider consulting a health-care professional for advice before embarking upon an exercise program.

The exercises recommended by the Health Promotion Units are swimming, walking and keep fit.

### Nourishment

In the past, it was thought that older people needed to eat a light diet of flavourless, steamed foods. However, eating too few calories means that the older person will be less able to cope with illness, injury or stressful situations.

Poor eating habits can be dangerous in old age, as an unbalanced diet can affect health and cause illness.

## Intellectual activities

As one grows older, it is very important to keep the brain active. Just as the body needs physical exercise to keep it supple, so too does the mind need intellectual stimulation to keep it active and alert. Board games, puzzles and crosswords are a good way of providing intellectual recreation. Games might include group games such as bingo or individual challenges such as chess or draughts. Using photographs and items from the past may help to stimulate memories and keep an older person's brain active.

Intellectual recreation can also include activities related to therapy. Intellectual activity could come from concentrating on painting, sewing or knitting.

### Safety, comfort and suitability

As with all the above physical and intellectual activities, issues connected with safety, comfort and suitability are of prime importance. If you are organising an event for the older service user there are aspects of health

    – Intellectual stimulation of the older person

    – Health and safety issues.

c) It is very important that you consider how you can involve the older person in planning the activity so as to empower them.

d) When you have carried out the chosen practical care task you must assess your own performance.

    – Did you achieve the aims that you set yourself?

    – Did you achieve the objectives of the practical care task?

    – Did you make the best use of available resources?

    – Did you meet the outcomes that you set for yourself?

    – Look at your own strengths – what did you do best?

    – What could you have done better?

    – How did you empower the service user?

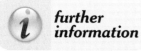

**further information**

Clarke L (2000) *Health and Social Care for Foundation GNVQ*. Nelson Thornes, Cheltenham

Clarke L (2000) *Health and Social Care for Intermediate GNVQ*. Nelson Thornes, Cheltenham

Clarke L (2002) *Health and Social Care GCSE*. Nelson Thornes, Cheltenham

Green S (2002) *BTEC National Early Years*. Nelson Thornes, Cheltenham

Nolan Y (1998) *Care. NVQ Level 2 Student Handbook*. Heinemann, Oxford

Nolan Y (2001) *Care. S/NVQ Level 3 Candidate Handbook*. Heinemann, Oxford

Stretch B (ed.) (2002) *BTEC National Health Studies*. Heinemann, Oxford

www.ageconcern.org.uk – Age Concern

www.arc.org.uk – Arthritis Research

www.asthma.org.uk – National Asthma Campaign

www.cpa.org.uk – Centre for Policy on Ageing

www.doh.gov.uk/kwkw – Keep warm, keep well

www.helptheaged.org.uk – Help the Aged

www.nhs.uk – NHS in UK

www.nos.org.uk – National Osteoporosis Society

## Summary

- People's health is affected by many factors, such as the time in which they are living, their ethnic group, their gender and their occupation.

- Older people still have physical, emotional, intellectual, social and cultural needs and these must be respected by carers.

- When older people are ill, they may be cared for and supported by a range of professionals, including community nurses, social workers, physiotherapists and GPs. There are also support groups such as Age Concern to help older people with dependent needs.

- Some more common adult illnesses such as hypothermia and osteoarthritis have telltale signs and symptoms that when recognised can be acted on to maximise effective care.

- There are set procedures for performing health checks such as measuring and recording pulse and body mass index.

# 7 Development and care of young children

## To complete this unit you will need to:

- Recognise the responsibilities of parenthood
- Describe milestones in physical development from birth to 3 years
- Describe milestones in intellectual development from birth to 3 years
- Describe the milestones of emotional and social development from birth to 3 years
- Review the care needs of a new baby
- Design a nursery for a new baby, evaluating its suitability.

 **AO1** Recognise the responsibilities of parenthood

### Preconceptual care

In the months before conception, a healthy lifestyle for the parents-to-be is important to ensure the development of a healthy baby.

A healthy lifestyle includes the following:

- A healthy diet
- Rest and exercise
- Avoiding diseases
- Avoiding certain substances
- Wearing the right clothing.

*Responsibilities of parenthood*

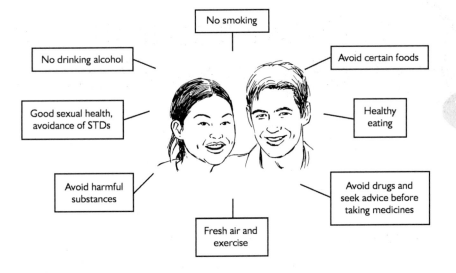

## Healthy diet

It is essential for the pregnant mother to eat a healthy diet as this lays the foundation for good health in later life. The pregnant mother should eat a well balanced diet.

### *The balance of good health*

*The nutrient triangle*

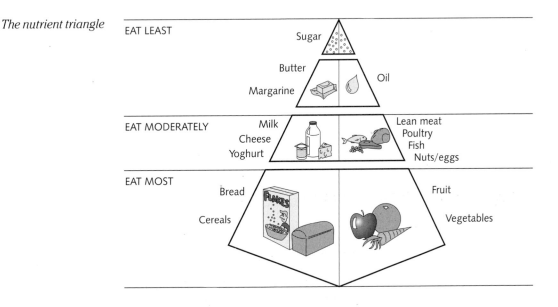

In 1994 the National Food Guide, *The Balance of Good Health* was published. It is based on the government's (MAFF) eight guidelines for a healthy diet. *The Balance of Good Health* is based upon five commonly accepted food groups, which are:

- Bread, other cereals and potatoes
- Meat fish and alternatives
- Fruit and vegetables

- Milk and dairy foods
- Fatty and sugary foods.

So, eat a variety of different foods to get a range of different nutrients. It is a good idea to keep the amount of sugar and fat consumed to within sensible recommended limits. Food such as cakes, biscuits, sweets and fizzy drinks contain sugar, which can make you put on weight while not supplying extra nutrients.

At the same time it is important to increase fresh fruit and vegetables and wholegrain cereals. Fresh fruit and vegetables supply vitamins but frozen vegetables must not be dismissed as they contain just as many vitamins and do not lose these during storage.

Cereals are important for fibre, which helps digestion and prevents constipation. Good fibre providers include wholegrain breakfast cereals, wholemeal bread and brown bread.

Pregnant women need to increase their protein intake slightly. You must have protein foods every day, including meat, fish, eggs, cheeses, pulse, textured vegetable proteins (TVP), nuts and Quorn. Calcium is vital for your baby's development and can be found in dairy foods such as cheese, milk and yogurt.

Folic acid is a vitamin B group vitamin, which is very important before and during pregnancy, especially in the first 12 weeks. It is advised that pregnant women take folic acid supplements to reduce the risk of spina bifida in their newborn baby. Good dietary sources of folic acid are fortified breakfast cereals, wholemeal bread, kidneys, brown rice, eggs and green leafy vegetables.

Iron is essential for a healthy blood supply for both mother and baby. Insufficient iron can lead to anaemia for the mother. Iron-rich foods include lean red meat, fortified breakfast cereals, oily fish, dried apricots,

## Case Study

Mandy is pregnant. Here is what she eats during a typical day:

**Breakfast**: Toast, black coffee with two sugars

**Snack**: Packet of crisps, fizzy sweet drink

**Lunch**: Sausage and chips, cup of tea

**Snack**: Bar of chocolate, fizzy drink

**Evening meal**: Cheese and tomato pizza and chips, cup of black coffee with two sugars

**During the evening**: Three cans of lager, three packets of crisps, packet of salted peanuts.

*Is this a healthy diet for a pregnant woman?*

green leafy vegetables, eggs and wholemeal bread. Fresh fruit and vegetables contain vitamin C, which is necessary for the body to absorb iron. Vitamin C is contained in blackcurrants, citrus fruit, sprouts, strawberries, etc.

## Exercise

Exercise has many benefits for both the mother and the unborn baby. It can help keep muscles and bones strong and promote good blood circulation, a healthy appetite and sound sleep.

*The benefits of exercise*

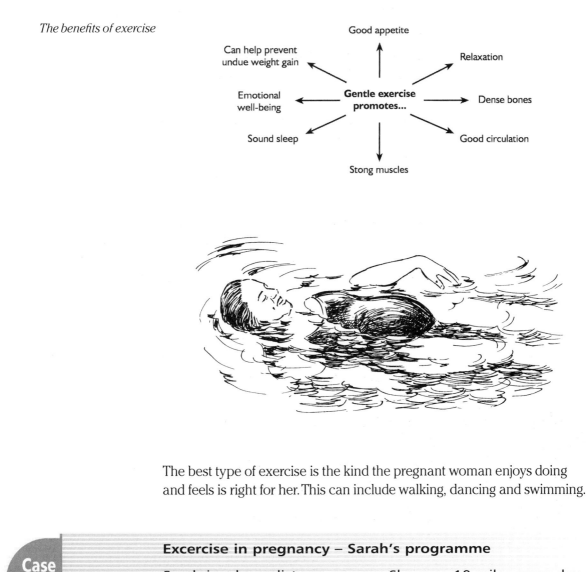

The best type of exercise is the kind the pregnant woman enjoys doing and feels is right for her. This can include walking, dancing and swimming.

**Case Study**

### Excercise in pregnancy – Sarah's programme

Sarah is a long distance runner. She runs 10 miles every day and does circuits four times a week at the gym. She is 3 months pregnant.

*Is her current exercise programme suitable for Sarah in the early stages of her pregnancy?*

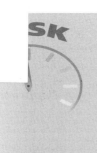

## Exercise in pregnancy – Sarah's programme

Draw up a suitable exercise programme for the rest of Sarah's pregnancy.

3 months:

4 months:

5 months:

6 months:

7 months:

8 months:

9 months:

## Clothing

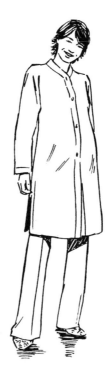

The body changes shape during pregnancy. The pregnant woman can wear loose clothing, particularly around the expanding waist. A larger, support-style bra with wide straps and adjustable fastening is advisable. Wearing shoes with low heels can help also as some women experience slight swelling in their feet.

## Emotions

Pregnancy is controlled by chemical substances called hormones. Hormones can also affect a woman's emotions.

Pregnant women can feel a variety of emotions from great happiness and excitement to anxiety and depression. Sometimes it can feel as if the pregnant woman is on an emotional roller-coaster.

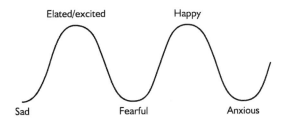

The pregnant woman will need lots of love, support and reassurance. These can be provided by the following:

- Baby's father
- Extended family
- Midwife
- GP
- Friends
- Hospital
- Antenatal class
- Birthing partner.

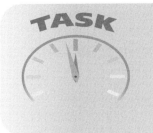

**TASK**

Working in a small group, can you think of how each of the above might provide emotional support for the pregnant woman?

## Physical changes

Pregnancy is a normal and natural process. The physical changes associated with pregnancy include:

- **Amenorrhoea (missing periods)** – this can also happen because of illness, shock, stress, severe weight loss and the menopause
- **Breast changes** – the breasts will become heavier and will 'tingle'; surface veins become visible and the nipple will become darker and more prominent
- **Nausea** – 'morning sickness' can occur at any time of the day or night
- **Frequent need to pass urine**
- **Weight gain** – slight weight gain at 8–9 weeks; after that weight gain becomes more significant.

*Screening in pregnancy*

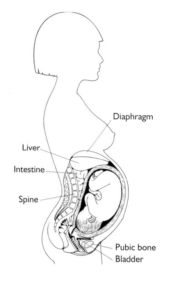

## The father's role

Both parents should be in good general health before attempting to have a baby. Preconceptual care means that fathers-to-be can also contribute to the formation of a healthy baby by following a healthy diet, giving up smoking and alcohol and avoiding harmful substances that can impair the quality of a man's sperm.

Advice on preconceptual care is available at doctors' surgeries and clinics. Depending on the family history of both partners, genetic counselling is sometimes offered. This means that the couple will be asked about inherited conditions in their families that might affect the health of their baby.

### Lifestyle

The lifestyle of both partners is important, whether before conception, during pregnancy or after the birth. Couples should be aware of any changes they could make for the well-being of their baby and decide if they are prepared to make the changes.

### How fathers feel

The father can feel left out, especially if he was not able to be present at the birth. Fathers need support and encouragement to become involved. They will gain confidence by holding, cuddling and caring for the baby. Fathers are entitled to paternity leave from work after the birth.

If they haven't already done so, both parents will need to discuss their roles and responsibilities towards the new and existing family members. Will they take it in turns to get up at night for the baby? Will the father take over some of the mother's responsibilities around the home while she cares for the new baby?

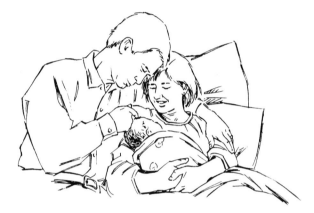

## Birthing partners

Do you think the father of the baby should be allowed into the delivery room?

If you are female, would you like your partner to be present during your delivery or would you prefer a different birthing partner, for example, your mother, friend or sister?

**AO2**

# Describe milestones in physical development from birth to 3 years

The growth and development of children is an incredible process. The newborn baby is helpless and totally dependent upon the mother and yet within a few years . . .

## Sequences in physical development

As children grow and develop a clear pattern or sequence of development emerges.

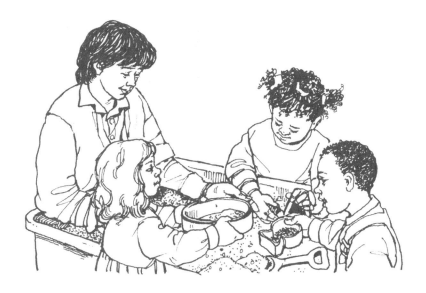

colour. Children playing in a sand pit, in a nursery, for example are learning about concepts such as mass and volume.

Children frequently ask very difficult questions the answers to which involve some very complicated concepts.

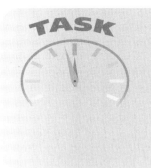

## Children's questions

Talk to mothers of small children and children themselves.

Write down some of the more difficult and sometimes amusing questions that children can ask. These questions can show the development of conceptual thought – e.g. child to mother: 'What keeps the sun up in the sky?'

Tables 7.4 and 7.5 outline the milestones in a child's intellectual development.

*Table 7.4  Intellectual development of an infant*

| Age | Intellectual development |
| --- | --- |
| Newborn babies | • Use their sense – sight, touch, taste, smell, hearing – to explore and experience their world<br>• Their reflexes, such as sucking and rooting, stimulate brain activity<br>• Crying when needing to be fed or changed is a way of communicating with the mother |
| 1 month | • Interested in sounds<br>• May recognise mother |

| 3 months | <ul><li>Recognises mother's face</li><li>Shows excitement</li><li>Listens, smiles</li><li>Holds a rattle by grasping</li><li>Takes an interest in surroundings</li></ul> |
|---|---|
| 6 months | <ul><li>Responds to speech by making noises (*vocalises*)</li><li>Uses eyes a lot</li><li>Holds toys</li><li>Explores using hands</li><li>Will show some understanding of the carer's voice, for example if the carer is happy or angry</li></ul> |
| 9 months | <ul><li>Tries to talk</li><li>May start to say DaDa</li><li>Shouts for attention</li><li>Understands 'No'</li><li>Can play 'peek a boo'</li><li>Can look for fallen toys</li><li>Have a memory of events such as bathtime and bedtime routines</li></ul> |
| 12 months | <ul><li>Knows own name</li><li>Has a vocabulary of about three words</li><li>Obeys simple instructions</li><li>Watches and copies adults</li><li>Repeats actions – such as dropping rattle</li><li>Knows what some objects are for, e.g. hairbrush, spoon</li></ul> |

*Table 7.5   Intellectual development: 1–3 years*

| Age | Intellectual development |
|---|---|
| 1.5 years | <ul><li>Uses 6–20 recognisable words</li><li>Repeats last word of short sentences</li><li>Enjoys and tries to join in with nursery rhymes</li><li>Picks up named toys</li><li>Enjoys looking at simple picture books</li><li>Builds a tower of three or four bricks</li><li>Scribbles and makes dots</li><li>Preference for right or left hand is shown</li></ul> |
| 2 years | <ul><li>Uses 50 or more recognisable words</li><li>Understands many more words</li><li>Puts two or three words together to form simple sentences</li><li>Refers to self by name</li><li>Asks names of objects and people</li><li>Scribbles in circles</li><li>Can build a tower of six or seven blocks</li><li>Hand preference is obvious and firmly established</li></ul> |

▶

| 2.5 years | • May use 200 words or more<br>• Knows full name<br>• Continually asking questions<br>• Likes stories and recognises self in photographs<br>• Builds a tower of seven or more blocks |
|---|---|
| 3 years | • States full name, sex and sometimes age<br>• Carries on simple conversations<br>• Constantly asks questions<br>• Demands favourite story over and over again<br>• Can count to 10 by rote<br>• Can thread wooden beads on string<br>• Can copy a circle and a cross<br>• Names colours<br>• Cuts up with scissors<br>• Paints with a large brush |

## TASK

### Milestones in development

Find out when a child that you know reached the following milestones:

● Said first word

● What was the first word

● Built a tower using three or more building blocks

● Made first scribble

● Knew own name

● Said first simple sentence

● Knew basic colours

● Said a nursery rhyme.

## Communication

It is important to understand that there is more to communication than using language. Babies communicate with other people before they can speak. Communication without using language, the spoken word, is called *non-verbal communication*.

*Non-verbal communication: how babies communicate*

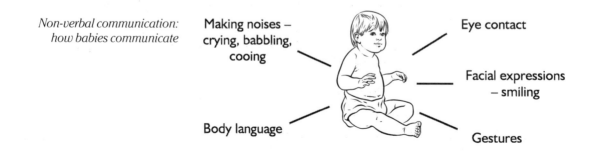

Making noises – crying, babbling, cooing

Eye contact

Facial expressions – smiling

Body language

Gestures

### How babies learn to talk

Babies learn to talk very early. This is called *verbal communication*. Humans are the only species that have the ability to use language. Language is an organised system of symbols that humans use to communicate and connect with the world and establish relationships with one another. The baby learns to talk by making sounds. These sounds are then put in order to shape recognisable words.

### Milestones in communication development

There are milestones in communication development.

First few weeks

- Baby makes some basic noises. These noises communicate to the mother the baby's needs, such as hunger, pain and distress.

Three months

- The baby makes 'cooing' sounds. The baby is practising the different sounds needed to make speech.

Six months

- The baby will make babbling sounds. Babbling is where the baby copies the speech rhythm of others.
- At the end of the first year, the child is adding different tone, pitch and rhythm into the pattern of sound. Mothers can often recognise some words.

Fifteen months

- The child will begin to say simple words and join in nursery rhymes.
- After this, the rate of language development is very fast. By the age of 3, children are fluent talkers. This is a remarkable achievement, especially when you consider how hard it is for adults to learn a foreign language.

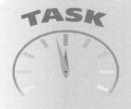

**TASK**

## Milestones in communication development

**Before you begin this activity, make sure that you seek the parents' permission.**

Divide your Health and Social Care group into three, each group to take one of the following:

- Baby 0–6 months
- Infant 7–12 months
- Toddler 15 months onward.

▶

7

Tape-record the communication noises and sounds of the child your group has chosen.

Using the information in the development chart above, work out which communication milestones have been reached.

Present your findings to the rest of the class.

### Ways of encouraging communication

A stimulating, caring environment where the child feels valued will actively promote good communication experiences.

Adults can promote effective communication by:

- Making eye contact and listening to the child
- Praising and encouraging the child to share ideas, thoughts and feelings
- Reading stories every day to the child
- Singing nursery rhymes with the child
- Making up stories with the child, encouraging the child to take the story further and develop ideas
- Being attentive
- Being patient
- Asking questions
- Providing opportunities where children can interact with others, both adults and children.

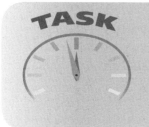

### TASK

### Promoting good communication

Using ICT, design, make and illustrate a book of nursery rhymes for children 2–3 years old.

### Barriers to communication

A barrier to communication is something that prevents effective communication taking place. Barriers to communication can be:

- Physical
- Emotional
- Cultural.

These are some of the reasons why children may find communication difficult:

- A physical problem – a lisp, a cleft palate
- Deafness – this may be either temporary or permanent
- Stammering – a common problem that occurs between the ages of 2 and 4 years old and in children who tend to think faster than they can speak
- A learning disability – Down's syndrome or autism
- Shyness
- More than one language being spoken at home – sometimes English is not the language usually spoken at home
- Poor stimulation – little opportunities to practice and develop communication, few toys and books.

The care worker will recognise the barriers to communication and can help the child to overcome them. This may mean referring the child to a speech therapist. Some care workers learn Makaton, and Sign Language communication can become established.

## AO4  Describe the milestones of emotional and social development from birth to 3 years

*Emotions* are feelings such as love, happiness, sadness, anger and joy. Young children can have very strong emotions and emotional development is about understanding, making sense of and exercising some control over these emotions.

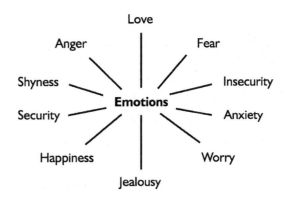

*Emotional development* is concerned with:

- The pattern of development of these feelings in children
- The way children express their feelings about themselves and their situation and understand what these feelings mean
- The feelings children have for other people such as friends, family members and carers.

Emotional and social development are very closely linked.

*Social development* means developing the skills that enable children to interact with other people in a meaningful and beneficial way. This process can sometimes be called *socialisation*.

Social development is concerned with:

- The ability to communicate and develop relationships with others
- The development of social skills such as sharing, observing rules and taking turns
- Socialisation – conforming to and accepting standards of behaviour, dress, hygiene and eating habits that are acceptable in society and do not offend others.

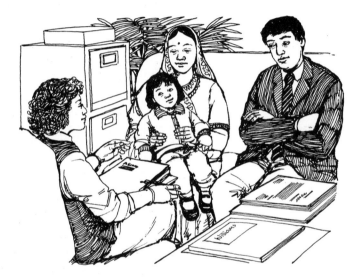

Today, Britain is a multicultural society.

Care workers recognise that different groups of people may observe their own set of customs. There are variations, for example, in forms of greeting, dress and eating habits.

Can you think of any other examples?

Emotional development is linked to all other areas of development, especially socialisation. Care workers need to take into account and understand fully the way a child develops emotionally and socially.

## Key features of development: birth to 1 year

As with other areas of development, a child's emotional and social development passes through different stages. This is called the sequence or pattern of development. The milestones that are reached are given an average age only and are meant as a guide. Health-care professionals and parents recognise also that each child is unique and develops in different areas at different rates.

The first year is crucial in terms of the baby's emotional and social development. It is important that babies form a strong bond with their mothers. Babies recognise their mother's smell and her voice and are comforted by her presence. Babies who form a strong bond with their mothers can often feel more confident about themselves when they come to socialise with others later. Babies play their part in this bonding process and they quickly learn that making eye contact, laughing and smiling helps to establish and maintain this contact with their mother.

*Table 7.6  Emotional and social development of an infant*

| Age | Emotional and social development |
| --- | --- |
| Birth to 1 month | • Babies use body movements to express pleasure, e.g. when being fed, when being bathed<br>• Enjoys feeding and cuddling |
| 1 month | • Cries in response to pain, hunger and thirst<br>• May sleep up to 20 hours in a 24-hour period<br>• Stops crying when picked up and spoken to<br>• Smiles in response to adults<br>• Turns to look at speaker's face |
| 3 months | • Enjoys being played with<br>• Misses carer and cries for him/her to return<br>• Responds happily to carer<br>• Becomes excited at prospect of a feed or bath<br>• Stays awake for longer periods of time |
| 6 months | • Can be anxious in the presence of strangers<br>• Can show anger and frustration<br>• Shows a clear preference for mother's company<br>• Puts everything in mouth<br>• Plays with hands and feet<br>• Tries to hold bottle when feeding<br>• Can be aware of the feelings of others, e.g. laugh if someone else laughs, cry if someone else cries |
| 9 months | • Can recognise individuals – mother, father, siblings<br>• Still anxious about strangers<br>• Sometimes irritable if routine is altered<br>• Plays 'peek-a-boo'<br>• Imitates hand-clapping<br>• Puts hand round cup when feeding |
| 12 months | • Shows affection<br>• Gives kisses and cuddles<br>• Likes to see familiar faces but less worried by strangers<br>• Drinks from a cup without assistance<br>• Holds a spoon but cannot feed him/herself<br>• Plays 'pat-a-cake'<br>• Quickly finds hidden toys |

## Environmental influences

The environment means the surroundings and conditions the child grows up in. The environment plays a significant role in the way children develop emotionally and socially. A happy, safe and secure environment where the child's needs are met in an atmosphere of love and care will help promote development.

The following conditions will help promote a positive environment where the child can grow emotionally and socially:

- A safe, secure and hygienic environment
- Equipment, books, toys, activities provided that match the needs of the child
- An atmosphere where the child is loved and nurtured and encouraged to progress
- Opportunities made available where children can express their individuality and experience independence
- Clear, appropriate behaviour standards established and reinforced
- Parents and carers who provide strong role models for children
- Strong, secure value base within the family unit.

## Bonds of affection

'Bonding' is the term given to the close relationship between the baby and the principal carer, usually the mother. This begins at birth and it is common practice now in hospitals for midwives to place the newborn baby on the mother's breast to help establish the bonding process.

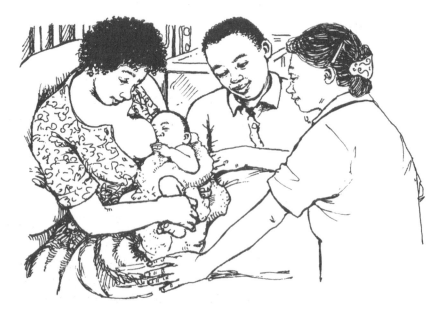

The love given by parents to the child is often called *unconditional love*, which means that the love they give to the child is without conditions and wanting anything back in return. Parents who love their children unconditionally accept them for who they are and not for what they want them to be. In the early days, the bonds of affection are strengthened by skin-to-skin contact and eye-to eye contact. The smell of the mother is also important to the baby. Love is one of the most basic needs of every human being.

## Shyness

Shyness is a recognised milestone in emotional and social development and clearly recognised by parents and carers. Shyness can be a useful protective response to unfamiliar people and situations. In these situations, carers can offer reassurance and comfort. Playing with other children and meeting adults in a safe, secure environment can help.

## Stress

Children can feel stress, just like adults. Stress can be triggered by events that are beyond a child's understanding. Here are some examples:

- Separation from mother or family member
- Starting nursery
- The birth of a new brother and sister
- Tension and rows at home
- Death in the family
- Moving home.

Crying, anxiety, temper tantrums, bed wetting and nightmares are all signs that a child is suffering from stress and that the child needs extra love and support.

## Security and insecurity

Security means feeling safe and loved. Insecurity means not feeling safe. Certain conditions can trigger feelings of insecurity such as too much discipline at home, or too little discipline. Insecure children can sometimes adopt challenging behaviour patterns and this is their way of letting the care worker know that something is wrong and that they need their help.

## Fears and nightmares

Children are very imaginative and their fears can seem very real to them. Children can be frightened of the dark, of monsters and of spiders, among other things. Children can also have nightmares and can wake up screaming and in an agitated state. It is important to reassure the child and gently help the child to go back to sleep.

*Table 7.7  Emotional and social development: 1–3 years*

| Age | Emotional development | Social development |
|-----|----------------------|-------------------|
| 1.5 years | • Affectionate, but may still be reserved with strangers<br>• Likes to see familiar faces | • Able to hold spoon and get food into mouth<br>• Holds drinking cup and hands it back when finished<br>• Can take off shoes and socks<br>• Bowel control may have been achieved<br>• Remembers where objects belong |
| 2 years | • Can display negative behaviour and resistance<br>• May have temper tantrums if thwarted<br>• Plays contentedly beside other children but not with them<br>• Constantly demands mother's attention | • Asks for food and drink<br>• Spoon feeds without spilling<br>• Puts on shoes |
| 2.5 years | • Usually active and restless<br>• Emotionally still very dependent on adults<br>• Tends not to want to share playthings | • Eats skilfully with a spoon and may sometimes use a fork<br>• Active and restless<br>• Often dry throughout the day |
| 3 years | • Becomes less prone to temper tantrums<br>• Affectionate and confiding, showing affection for siblings<br>• Begins to understand sharing | • Eats with a fork and a spoon<br>• May be dry throughout the night |

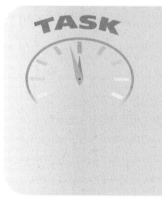

**TASK**

## Milestones in social development

Interview the mother of a toddler or a small child.

Try to find out what age her child reached the following milestones in emotional and social development:

- Puts on shoes
- Eats with a spoon
- Potty-trained
- Shares toys with others
- Likes to see familiar faces.

## Self-esteem

Self-esteem is about the feelings we have about ourselves.

The expressions self-concept and self-esteem are often used by health care professionals.

Self-esteem is based upon the judgement of others of ourselves and upon our own judgement. If we are happy about ourselves, we will have high

*Who am I? What am I like?*
*Do I like who I am?*

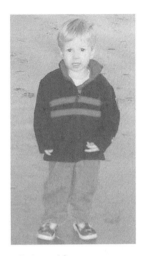

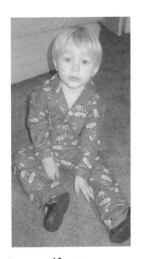

High self-esteem

Low self-esteem

Praise
Learning new skills
+ Expression of feelings
Independence
= **High self-esteem**

Poor relationships
Too much discipline
— Little pride in self
Unsure about physical appearance
= **Low self-esteem**

self-esteem. If we are unhappy and do not like ourselves, we will have low self-esteem and little confidence.

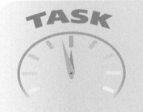

### Praising children

You are a care worker in a nursery. Design some stickers to praise the children.

## Role of play in development

Play is the natural way that children learn and discover about themselves and the world they live in.

Play encourages all areas of development, physical, intellectual, emotional and social. Language is also developed through play.

There are several types of play:

- Solitary play
- Parallel play
- Looking-on play
- Joining-in play
- Co-operative play.

Care workers acknowledge the different types of play and provide plenty of opportunities for children to develop a range of skills.

**Solitary play**
*0–2 years*
*Child plays alone, adult nearby*

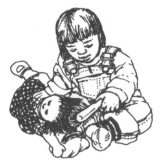

**Parallel play**
*2–3 years*
*Children play alongside each
other but do not play together*

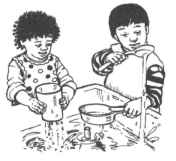

**Looking-on play**
*Child on the outside, looking in
Becoming ready to join in
and play with others*

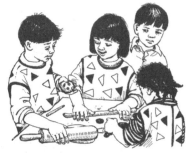

**Joining-in play**
*Children join with others to
play and watch and copy
each other*

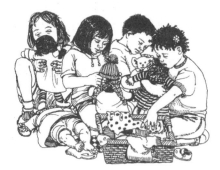

**Co-operative play**
*Children playing together
Sharing decisions about
what to play and who does what*

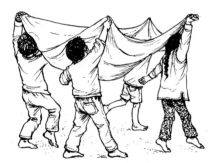

**AO5** | **Review the care needs of a new baby**

## Postnatal care

Postnatal care means care of the mother and baby after birth (*post* = after, *natal* = birth).

There are three professionals who look after the baby and mother after birth:

- The midwife
- The health visitor
- The doctor.

### The midwife

The midwife visits the mother at home until the baby is at least 10 days old.

### The health visitor

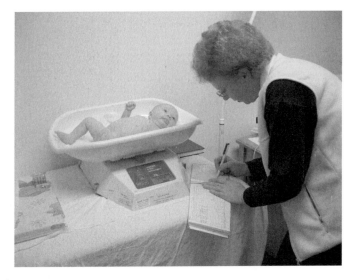

The health visitor will visit the mother at home but the mother can also visit her local baby clinic after that.

### The doctor

The doctor (paediatrician) will physically examine the mother and baby to check that both are healthy.

## Role of professionals

The midwife and health visitor will:

- Help and advise the mother on feeding the baby
- Check that the mother and baby are both in good health and offer support

- Check that the baby is making normal progress
- Weigh the baby regularly to check progress is being made
- Offer advice on immunisation
- Offer advice on health and safety
- Let the mother know about the clinic and when she should attend; there she can also meet other mothers and share experiences
- Talk to the new mother about how she is feeling emotionally.

Both the midwife and the health visitor will make physical checks on the baby to see that the umbilical cord has been cleaned thoroughly. The umbilical cord shrivels and drops off within 7–10 days.

The doctor will:

- Examine the baby and carry out neonatal (new born) screening tests
- Examine the mother to check that all stages of pregnancy have been completed satisfactorily.

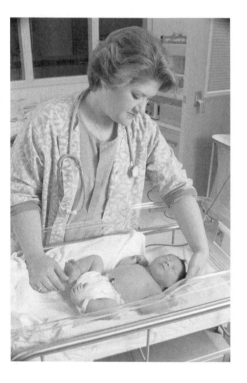

## Formalities after the birth

- The midwife and a specialist doctor will check the baby, if the birth takes place in hospital
- The main checks include breathing, heartbeat and response to stimuli, as well as weight, length and head circumference
- A special identity bracelet is attached to the baby in hospitals
- The baby is washed and dressed

- The mother is checked, made comfortable and given time to rest
- Parents are given time to be with the baby
- The baby may be given a breast-feed
- The baby is allowed to sleep and recover.

## Tests for baby

### PKU test

Phenylketonuria (PKU) is very rare and occurs when the baby's body cannot use a chemical found in milk. A few pinpricks of blood are taken from the baby's heel and tested. A special diet can correct the condition.

### Cystic fibrosis

This is a disorder that causes lung disease and specialist help is available.

### Congenital dislocation of the hip

The hip joints are tested to see if they are flexed properly. If the hip is dislocated, treatment will be given.

### Thyroid deficiency test

The thyroid is found in the throat. A child's physical and intellectual development can be slowed down if the thyroid is not working properly. Treatment is given using *thyroxine*, the thyroid hormone.

*The new baby*

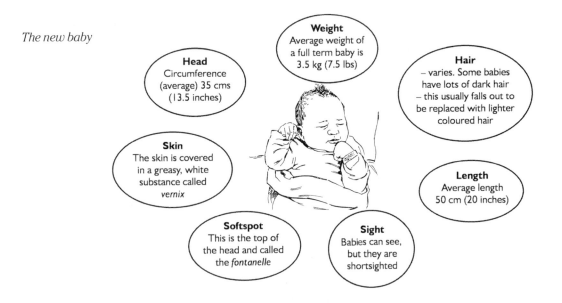

**Weight**
Average weight of a full term baby is 3.5 kg (7.5 lbs)

**Head**
Circumference (average) 35 cms (13.5 inches)

**Hair**
– varies. Some babies have lots of dark hair – this usually falls out to be replaced with lighter coloured hair

**Skin**
The skin is covered in a greasy, white substance called *vernix*

**Length**
Average length 50 cm (20 inches)

**Softspot**
This is the top of the head and called the *fontanelle*

**Sight**
Babies can see, but they are shortsighted

## Tests for the mother

The mother will be examined to see if the uterus is returning to normal after the delivery of the baby. At around 6 weeks after the birth, the mother has a postnatal examination. This is usually carried out by the family

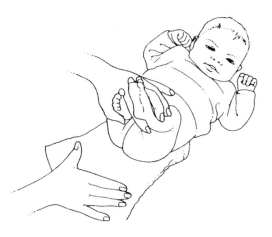

nappies and these can be bought at most large stores. They can be expensive but for busy mothers they are more convenient.

## TASK

### The advantages and disadvantages of terry-towelling and disposable nappies

Can you think of any advantages and disadvantages of buying:

● Terry towelling cotton nappies?

● Disposable nappies?

| Cotton nappies | Disposable nappies |
|---|---|
| Advantages | Advantages |
| | |
| Disadvantages | Disadvantages |
| | |

Work out the average cost of using disposable nappies and then towelling nappies on a baby for one year.

### *Nappy rash*

Nappy rash is when the skin becomes red and sore around the baby's bottom. Sometimes, if left untreated, a rash can develop. Nappy rash is caused by ammonia, which is produced when urine comes into contact with germs. Germs are present in the stools (faeces) that the baby has passed and can also be present in the nappy if it is not cleaned properly.

To help prevent nappy rash:

● Change the nappy frequently

● Sterilise and wash towelling nappies thoroughly

- Use a nappy cream such as zinc and castor oil cream or lotion to help protect the baby's skin
- Use nappy liners – these are disposable
- Leave off the nappy as much as possible
- Seek medical advice if the sores do not heal up.

### Protecting the baby through parent cleanliness

It is not always possible to keep a baby spotlessly clean nor is it always a good idea. A child's immune system needs to develop and exposure to some germs is normal. It is impossible to create and maintain a germ-free environment in the home. Nevertheless, parents should try to keep the baby's skin, nappy, clothes, blankets, toys and equipment clean so that germs and bacteria do not multiply.

It is important that parents protect their baby from infection by following certain hygiene rules:

- Always wash hands after going to the toilet, before making up a feed, before and after changing a nappy and before feeding a baby. If breast feeding, the breast and nipple should be thoroughly cleansed regularly and breast pads changed frequently.
- Clean feeding bottles after every feed. There are sterilising kits to help with this.
- Wash baby clothes and bedding frequently at the appropriate temperature.
- Wash toys such as rattles and soft teddy-bear toys regularly.

### Bathtime

Preparation

- Assemble everything you need within easy reach: baby bath filled with warm water, test the temperature with elbow (37°C), cotton wool, changing mat, two warm baby towels, clean nappy, cream, brush and comb, clothes, lidded bucket for soiled nappy, baby soap
- Make sure that the room is warm, not less than 20°C (68°F), and that there are no draughts
- Wash your hands before bathing baby – make sure nails are short.

Preparation

**Bathtime Routine**

- Never leave the baby alone
- Undress baby, leaving the nappy on, wrap in warm baby towel
- Clean the face using damp cotton wool and water

## Summary

- Correct diet and exercise play a major role in the health of a mother and her unborn baby.

- Milestones in the physical development of children from birth to 3 years include being able to lift the head and being able to walk without assistance.

- Milestones in the intellectual development of children from birth to 3 years include learning to talk, scribbling with pens and increasing memory.

- Milestones in the emotional and social development from birth to 3 years include being reserved with strangers but not with known people, remembering where toys need to be put away and beginning to understand sharing.

- Postnatal care involves looking after the mother and the baby. It includes various health checks on both just after the birth and ongoing care to ensure, for example, that the baby is bathed properly and that nappies are changed regularly.

- A baby's nursery should be carefully designed and fitted with appropriate and safe equipment.

# Preparing to work with young children

## 8

## To complete this unit you will need to:

- Identify the different types of care and education provision for young children and how it meets their needs
- Describe job roles and the skills and qualities required when working with children
- Recognise how to promote and maintain a safe environment for young children
- Investigate how the role of play contributes to the development of the child
- Design a suitable layout for a care and education setting for young children
- Plan and carry out an activity to intellectually stimulate young children and evaluate the success of the activity.

**AO1** Identify the different types of care and education provision for young children and how it meets their needs

Young children can be looked after by a wide variety of people.

### Childminder

Childminding is the most popular form of daycare for working parents, with more than 300,000 children in England and Wales cared for by registered childminders. Registered childminders, who are self-employed, work in their own homes to care for other people's children. Unlike nannies and au pairs, they must be registered with their local Social Services Department and have their work premises inspected regularly.

spent in the normal nursery session. Breakfast, lunch and tea are provided. 'Wrap around care' is run by a private provider, and clients pay for this service. The tax credit system can be used for this.

## Safety and protection

Children are vulnerable and young children have no understanding of danger, so it is up to parents and carers to ensure their safety at all times. As children develop, they need to explore their world and their environment. Carers need to take measures to reduce hazards but they must be careful not to over-protect children, as they need to gain confidence.

**Case Study**

You are a student nursery nurse, working with 3–5-year-olds.

During a home corner play session, you notice that Lee has smacked Jack with a wooden spoon. You stop Lee to talk to him about what is happening. He tells you that his Daddy hits him with a piece of wood, and shows you severe bruising on both legs.

*What would you do to help this little boy?*

*Find out from the nursery manager about the correct procedures for dealing with child protection issues.*

## Health

Everyone wants to be healthy. It is easy to take being healthy for granted, until something goes wrong and we become ill.

'Health' comes from an Old English word meaning 'whole', and the term includes physical, emotional, intellectual and social well-being. Health and well-being should mean that a person feels positively well and is not just free of disease or illness. It is difficult to define and collect information about 'well-being', as it often relates to how individual people feel about themselves and their personal experiences. Well-being is harder to define than illness, as it is often taken for granted. To make it clearer, there are three ways of looking at health and well-being:

- A negative way of looking at health and well-being can be to look at it as the absence of any physical illness, disease or mental distress. This definition is saying that a person has done nothing to contribute to this healthy state.

- A more positive way of looking at health and well-being is to say that a person achieves a healthy state through becoming and staying physically fit and mentally healthy. This means that the person contributes to their own well-being through keeping healthy and fit.

- The 'holistic way' of looking at health and well-being is when physical, social, intellectual and emotional factors are all seen to contribute to the health of the individual.

People's basic health needs do not change. The differences are in the ability of each person to provide for his or her own needs. In other words, people need different amounts and types of support to meet their needs throughout life.

*Basic health needs of individuals*

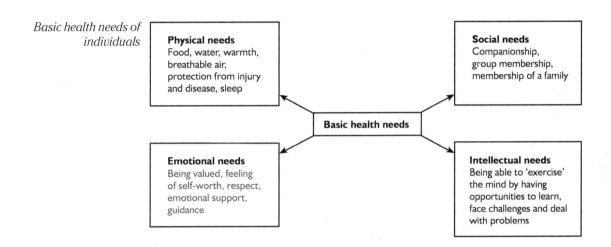

**Physical needs**
Food, water, warmth, breathable air, protection from injury and disease, sleep

**Social needs**
Companionship, group membership, membership of a family

**Basic health needs**

**Emotional needs**
Being valued, feeling of self-worth, respect, emotional support, guidance

**Intellectual needs**
Being able to 'exercise' the mind by having opportunities to learn, face challenges and deal with problems

Different needs also have differing importance:

- Food, water and shelter – basic human physical needs – are essential to stay alive
- The next most important need is safety
- Having achieved the first two needs, a person is in need of emotional and social support. Only when all these needs have been met is it realistic to consider needs for self-respect and self-esteem and, finally, personal fulfilment.

For example, people who are starving may take risks, which could affect their health and well-being, in order to obtain food, or may be prepared to degrade themselves by doing things they would not do if they were fully fed. The primary need of starving people is for food and only later can they consider their self-respect.

In addition to these factors, increasing attention is being paid to lifestyle factors. Why do cancer, heart disease and stroke occur most commonly in Western society? The quest to find out is known as *epidemiology*. Epidemiologists are now identifying lifestyle factors, particularly diet and lack of exercise, as causes of health problems. We all therefore have the power to influence our own health and that of our family.

## Hygiene

It is essential that a rigorous hygiene routine is established from the beginning. Later, as the child grows, personal hygiene skills should be encouraged so that by the time the child reaches nursery school s/he can independently care for skin, hair, nails and teeth at a basic level. Children must learn that lack of hygiene can lead to infections and disease, and is socially unacceptable.

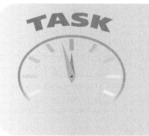

### Hygiene education

Without using words, make brightly coloured, attractive pictures to display near the wash basins in a nursery, showing children the correct way to wash their hands.

It is important to remember the difference between the terms 'growth' and 'development':

● Growth refers to an increase in actual size of a person – in other words, their physical growth

● Development means a person's increasing ability to master more complex skills, for example a child's ability to walk, talk or manipulate things with the fingers.

Becoming taller is an obvious growth, while a baby's ability to reach for objects or transfer them from one hand to another shows a development of complex skills.

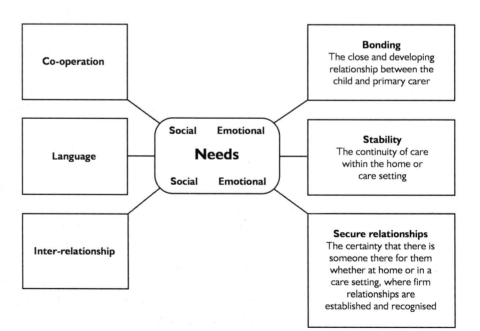

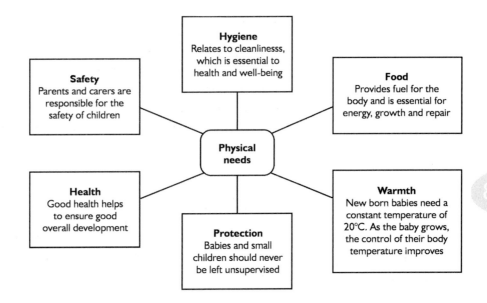

## Food

In order to grow properly a child must have a balanced diet, consisting of the major nutrients. There are five groups of nutrients: proteins, carbohydrates, fats, vitamins and minerals. Food and nutrition for babies and children is covered in detail in Unit 12.

## Warmth

The body needs a certain body temperature in order to survive. The heat regulation system is stored in the part of the brain called the *hypothalamus*. Shivering is the body's response to cold; tiny muscles move under the skin to generate heat. Sweating is the body's response to overheating; when the body overheats, blood rushes to the surface of the skin, which induces sweating, thereby cooling the body down. Adults and older children know when they are cold, and can warm up by eating warm food and/or drink, exercising, adding extra layers of clothes and even turning up the heat on the central heating thermostat. Carers must be aware that babies and small children need to have the temperature of their environment regulated in order to maintain their comfort in hot and cold weather.

## Bonding

Children have an inbuilt need to form a strong, stable relationship with their primary carer. The primary carer is often the mother, but this role can be filled by the father, or the main person who is looking after the child. Bonding is critical to the child's social and emotional development. Bonding provides the child with a sense of trust, familiarity and continuity in their first relationship. If children have a secure relationship with their primary carer their trust and self confidence will grow, enabling them to form wider relationships.

## Stability

Stable or secure relationships and surroundings are fundamental to the idea of stability. Children need routine, and carers should always help children to understand what is happening to them and why. It is important to handle changes in their routine sensitively, as these can be upsetting and unsettling. Familiar toys can offer security and comfort to a child. Firm rules and consistent boundaries contribute to the child's sense of stability.

## Secure relationships

If secure relationships are in place, the child will develop to find his/her full potential.

### Family relationships

How early are relationships formed? The answer is early! No one really knows how early a baby notices its mother, father or main carer; the important point is that, if a child is denied positive early relationships for a long time, this will affect the child's development. Babies who are neglected or ill-treated, who have had little stimulation, eye contact or physical contact, need a lot of help to become bright and affectionate themselves. Similarly, as the child grows, the relationship that develops gives the child a pattern for future relationships.

### The influence of parents

Influential psychologists, such as Freud, Bowlby and Piaget, said that a child's early relationship with its parents (particularly the mother) sets the tone of later relationships. Children who have secure relationships with their parents are more likely to be accepted by their peers (meaning their friends and contemporaries). Sometimes children who have difficult relationships with brothers and sisters form closer friendships outside the home.

### Nature and nurture

Parenting is a two-way process. It would be easy for parents if their children simply followed whatever their parents wanted them to do. Children, however, have personalities and wills of their own so being a parent is an *interactive*, or two-way, process. Two children in the same family can be very different even if their parents have brought them up in roughly the same way.

### The influence of the family

Although the relationship between parent or main carer and child is a central one, other early relationships soon become significant. The relationship between brothers and sisters may be tempestuous at times but they also provide many positive factors in the development of children.

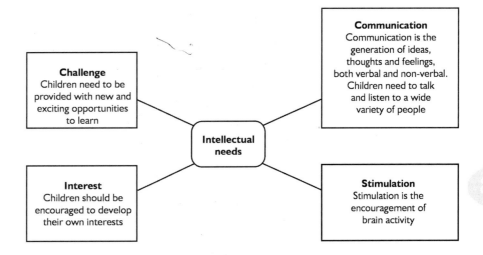

**Challenge**
Children need to be provided with new and exciting opportunities to learn

**Communication**
Communication is the generation of ideas, thoughts and feelings, both verbal and non-verbal. Children need to talk and listen to a wide variety of people

**Intellectual needs**

**Interest**
Children should be encouraged to develop their own interests

**Stimulation**
Stimulation is the encouragement of brain activity

## Communication

The need to communicate is essential to all human beings. From the moment of birth babies cry to communicate their needs to their carers. They continue to do this during their first year of life. Communicating with babies and young children is one of the most important roles of primary carers and early-years workers. They must recognise that children need plenty of opportunities to experiment with and use language, and to develop their communication skills.

## Stimulation

Stimulation is essential if babies and young children are to develop to their full potential intellectually. Stimulation begins at birth with contact with the mother. The environment can also provide a rich source of stimulation. A child who is denied stimulation can fail to thrive in all the key areas of development – intellectual, social, emotional and physical. The care worker has to recognise that each child is an individual and needs to explore at his/her own pace. Too much stimulation can be just as bad as too little, as the child can become overexcited and irritable.

### Interest

Children are all different and, as a result, have different needs and interests. Therefore it is very important for primary carers and care workers to provide toys and games that will stimulate the children's interests. Interests can be developed by arranging suitable visits and activities.

## Developing children's interests

Think about a young child (age 1–5). Make a list of all his/her interests. Plan a range of activities that would develop each interest.

### Challenge

Challenge is essential for intellectual growth. It should involve taking children beyond what they know and can do now. Exploration is vital, but carers must ensure that the challenging environment is also a safe environment. In this way children's intellectual development can be accelerated.

## Social Needs

Care provision for young children also provides for their social needs.

Children learn to socialise and co-operate with others in groups. Children learn how to co-operate by copying other people or copying other children in the care setting. Peer pressure also plays a part in their development of these skills. The child learns to co-operate in care settings by learning basic patterns of behaviour. They will learn how to behave in a wide range of settings, how to expect others to behave, and create inter-relationships. Hopefully they will perceive the care setting as structured and predictable and therefore have a feeling of security in which they can experiment with different behaviours. These will lay the foundation for the future development of the child.

Language is the main way that children communicate. Language is learned, and the child's ability to operate within society, family and care settings is affected by their ability to use language effectively.

In care settings children can use their skills (non-verbal, listening, written and spoken) to further develop the language skills already learned within their family and wider community.

**AO2** ## Describe job roles and the skills and qualities required when working with children

All care workers need to have the skills and qualities illustrated below and on page 247.

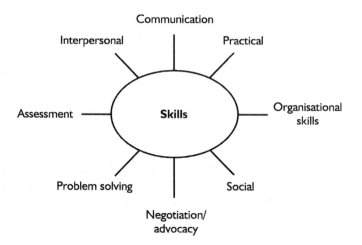

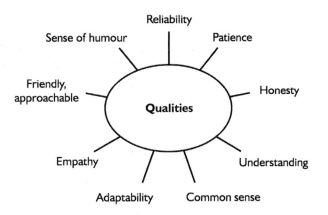

A *skill* is a special quality acquired by training and practice. Early-years workers, in their everyday work, will need to draw upon a wide range of skills.

*Interpersonal skills* involve relating to other people. Communication is an important part of this process. Sometimes, the early-years worker will need to speak on behalf of a child or a child's family. This is called *advocacy*. Meeting and sharing information with parents, carers and other professionals will allow social skills to be practised.

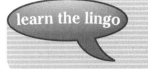

**Advocacy** means speaking to other professionals on behalf of a child or their family.

Practical skills involve the demonstration of a 'hands on' approach to any situation that may occur. Because early years children take part in a lot of practical activities, it is useful for the care worker to organise time, space and resources.

The assessment of individual children's needs is part of recognising the individuality of children. *Problem-solving* is having the ability to respond to situations and problems as and when they occur.

A *quality* is a personal attribute or feature and, as such, is an expression of personality and temperament. Early-years workers need to be reliable, as children are dependent on them to meet their needs. Patience and a sense of humour are also desirable qualities, as sometimes caring for others can be demanding and challenging, and it is helpful if the worker can be understanding and show empathy for the child in their care. Sorting out problems often demands common sense and the child must be able to approach the early-years worker for help and support. As workers have access to personal information and belongings they must also be scrupulously honest.

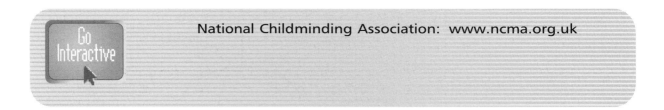

National Childminding Association: www.ncma.org.uk

## Job roles

### *Nursery nurse*

Nursery nurses care for children from birth to school age. Their job can involve many care tasks, including washing, toileting, changing clothing, feeding and playing. An important part of their job involves planning for learning activities and play following the guidelines set out in the Early Learning goals. These goals were published in October 1999 and, although not a curriculum in themselves, nevertheless establish expectations for most children to reach.

Nursery nurses can work in a variety of settings from working privately for a family to working in hospitals, infant and nursery schools, residential homes for the disabled, crèches, etc.

#### Qualifications

The special skills required for this type of care are recognised and nursery nurses have either a CACHE diploma or an OCR/Btec National diploma or certificate in Health, Social Care and Early Years.

NVQs in Early Years and Education at levels 2 or 3 are also available for nursery nurses.

### *Playgroup leader*

Play workers are part of a team that provides opportunities for children from 5–15 to play in different ways and different settings. They find different ways to stimulate children through play. Play workers use their expertise to provide a safe and creative environment provided with a wide range of materials and equipment. Play workers provide opportunities for both indoor and outdoor play. Indoor activities can include arts and crafts, music, drama, story-telling, baking, counting and measuring, etc. Outdoor play can include climbing, digging, riding a bike, playing tag, rounders and other ball games.

Recently there has been a massive upsurge in demand for childcare, with the result that there are plenty of employment opportunities in this sector.

#### Qualifications

There is a national framework of training that will lead to qualifications in this area. They can include the following:

- NVQ in Playwork level 2 & 3
- Modern apprenticeship
- Higher education courses, e.g. Diploma and Certificate in Playwork
- Playwork Foundation Course.

### Childminder

Childminding involves looking after other people's children in your own home. Childminders must be registered with the local Social Services Department before they start to look after someone else's child. There are stringent legal requirements to be met, including restrictions on the number of children to be minded in your home at any one time. A safety audit will be conducted on your home and you will require an Enhanced Police Disclosure. Health records are also checked. The childminder's home is visited on an annual basis to ensure that standards are being met.

Childminders are self-employed and negotiate their own fees and contracts with the parents. This is a way of earning money while looking after your own child. Childminding is an important and responsible job, and requires people who enjoy looking after children and are concerned for their welfare.

Qualifications
- No formal qualifications are needed
- Childminders may wish to be assessed for NVQs in Early Years Care and Education
- CACHE Certificate in Childminding Practice
- CCP Certificate in Childminding Practice – Nationally accredited qualification.

### Nursery teacher

Most nursery classes or units attached to schools have a designated person in charge. This is often the nursery teacher. The main function of nursery classes is to educate, although they are also caring for the children. A nursery teacher will plan and deliver the curriculum for the Foundation Stage. The Foundation Stage curriculum sets early learning goals to be reached by the time children enter Year 1 of primary school. The early learning goals consist of:

- Personal, social and educational development
- Communication, language and literacy
- Mathematics
- Knowledge and understanding of the world
- Physical development
- Creative development.

Qualifications

This is a degree entry profession.

## Early years care values

Early years care values underpin all aspects of child-care provision. The following are the early years care values:

- Welfare of the child
- Maintaining a healthy and safe environment
- Working with others
- Helping the child to meet its full potential
- Valuing diversity
- Equality of opportunity
- Anti-discrimination
- Confidentiality
- The reflective practitioner.

### Welfare of the child

When working with children, the care worker must recognise that the health, happiness and well-being of the child are most important. All early-years workers must give priority to the rights and well-being of the children they work with. Children must be listened to and their views and worries taken seriously.

### Maintaining a healthy and safe environment

At all times the child-care environment should be safe and secure. In addition, to comply with any local authority regulations, all child-care settings will have a health and safety policy that will include:

- Procedures for using equipment
- Policies for dealing with spills of bodily fluids
- Clear safety rules for children's conduct
- Stringent safety precautions, e.g. non-slip surfaces, safety glass, doors with safety catches
- Procedures for staff to report potential hazards
- Policies for collecting children
- Clear rules to ensure that staff practise safety, e.g. keeping hot drinks away from children
- Any adult working with children has a responsibility to protect children from abuse.

## Working with others

This can be:

- Working in partnership with parents/families
- Working with other professionals.

### Working in partnership with parents/families

Parents and families play a key role in their children's lives and are therefore knowledgeable about their children, so their views should be listened to and respected. Working in partnership with parents is recognised as being of major value and importance.

### Working with others

Working as part of a team is recognised as good practice. This may be a multi-disciplinary team with representation from other colleagues and relevant agencies such as Social Services. Those who work as nannies or childminders may find it helpful to see themselves as part of a team together with the child's family. Working in partnership with parents is recognised as being of major value and importance.

## Helping the child to meet its full potential

The early years are a time of rapid learning. It is vital to recognise that learning begins at birth and that this early learning lays down foundations for future growth and development. Children should be offered a wide range of experiences and learning opportunities that will support and enhance all areas of their development. High expectations should be set for all children. Play is a central and valuable part of young children's learning. Records concerning their children should be shared with parents.

## Valuing diversity

Valuing diversity means appreciating difference. Britain today is multi-cultural and we recognise the richness and diversity that different cultures bring to our society.

## Equality of opportunity

All children are individuals with different needs and should not be treated the same. All children should be treated with 'equal concern'. The support and help offered to children should meet their individual needs in order to provide equality of opportunity.

## Anti-discrimination

Discrimination describes how one person treats another person or group unfairly, based on prejudice. Early years workers must not discriminate on the grounds of gender, racial origin, disability, sexuality, or cultural or social background.

### Confidentiality

Confidentiality is a principle common to all health, social-care and early-years services. This means that, before any information you have about a service user is shared with other people, the service user's permission must be obtained.

There are certain times when service user confidentiality has to be limited:

- If the service user is a danger to themselves or others
- If they are unconscious and cannot give information about their medical condition
- If they are about to commit or have committed a crime
- If a court of law (not the police) requests information
- If any kind of abuse has taken or is about to take place.

### The reflective practitioner

Early-years workers should think about their own professional performance so that they can improve and develop their own good practice. Workers can also seek advice from other professionals to extend their expertise and knowledge.

## AO3 Recognise how to promote and maintain a safe environment for young children

### Responsibilities in protecting children from harm

Children are vulnerable to accidents and hazards, so parents and carers need to make safe and supervise their environment. Children do need to explore by seeing, touching and by doing. This helps them to gain in confidence. Children need constant supervision, but carers must recognise that some activities are more dangerous than others.

In a nursery setting there will be a designated member of staff with the responsibility for health and safety. They will also promote awareness of health and safety issues to all staff, children and parents. Policy documents relating to health and safety must be in place and must be reviewed regularly.

### Identification of hazards

Hazards are all around us and care workers must realise that it is part of their role to identify dangers in their place of work. We will examine two areas in detail:

- Nursery setting see figure on page 253
- Home setting see figure on page 254.

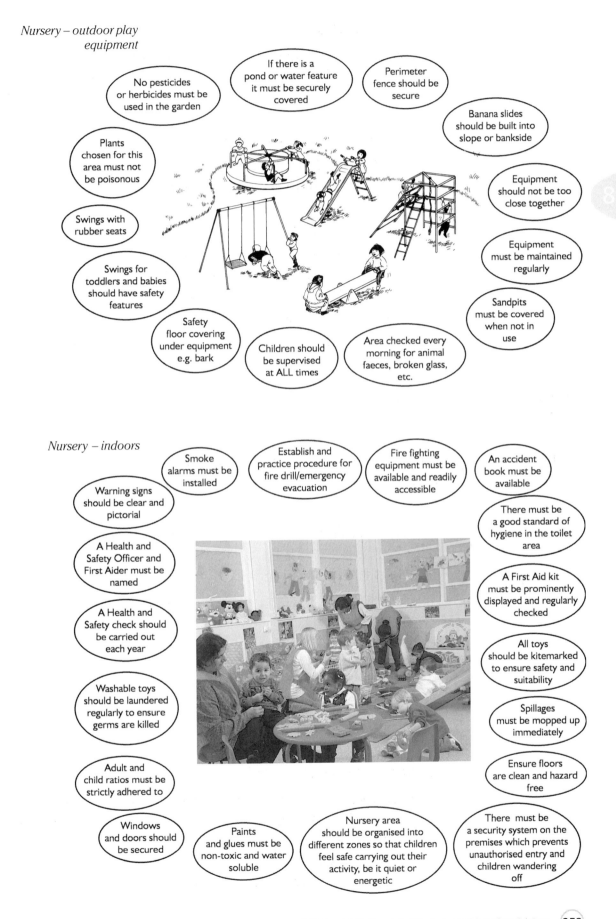

*Nursery – outdoor play equipment*

No pesticides or herbicides must be used in the garden

If there is a pond or water feature it must be securely covered

Perimeter fence should be secure

Banana slides should be built into slope or bankside

Plants chosen for this area must not be poisonous

Equipment should not be too close together

Swings with rubber seats

Equipment must be maintained regularly

Swings for toddlers and babies should have safety features

Sandpits must be covered when not in use

Safety floor covering under equipment e.g. bark

Children should be supervised at ALL times

Area checked every morning for animal faeces, broken glass, etc.

*Nursery – indoors*

Smoke alarms must be installed

Establish and practice procedure for fire drill/emergency evacuation

Fire fighting equipment must be available and readily accessible

An accident book must be available

Warning signs should be clear and pictorial

There must be a good standard of hygiene in the toilet area

A Health and Safety Officer and First Aider must be named

A First Aid kit must be prominently displayed and regularly checked

A Health and Safety check should be carried out each year

All toys should be kitemarked to ensure safety and suitability

Washable toys should be laundered regularly to ensure germs are killed

Spillages must be mopped up immediately

Adult and child ratios must be strictly adhered to

Ensure floors are clean and hazard free

Windows and doors should be secured

Paints and glues must be non-toxic and water soluble

Nursery area should be organised into different zones so that children feel safe carrying out their activity, be it quiet or energetic

There must be a security system on the premises which prevents unauthorised entry and children wandering off

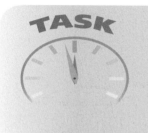

## Dangerous activities

Categorise the activities in the list below, using a star rating system, as follows:

***** Very dangerous
**** Dangerous
*** Moderately dangerous
** Little or low danger
* Minimal danger.

- Sandpit play
- Paddling pool
- Painting
- Wendy house
- Clay/dough play

- Baking
- Pretend play
- Cutting out shapes
- Bathing a doll
- Digging/planting

- Climbing frame
- Reading
- Banana slide
- Swing
- Feeding a pet

*Home setting*

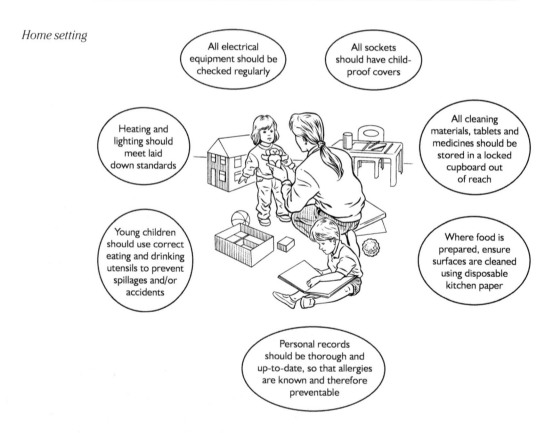

All electrical equipment should be checked regularly

All sockets should have child-proof covers

Heating and lighting should meet laid down standards

All cleaning materials, tablets and medicines should be stored in a locked cupboard out of reach

Young children should use correct eating and drinking utensils to prevent spillages and/or accidents

Where food is prepared, ensure surfaces are cleaned using disposable kitchen paper

Personal records should be thorough and up-to-date, so that allergies are known and therefore preventable

## Reporting of hazards

All care settings must have systems in place for the reporting and recording of all hazards and accidents. There are many ways of doing this, including:

- Accident report book

- Risk assessment (hazard audit)
- Vertical reporting to line manager.

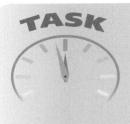

## Safe working systems – a checklist

- Do you know who your supervisor is?
- Who do you report accidents and hazards to?
- Do you know the safe way of doing your job?
- Have you been instructed in the use and limitations of any equipment you are using?
- Has anyone assessed whether the equipment you are using is safe for the job?
- If things go wrong, do you know what to do?
- Are you aware of a system for checking that tasks you are asked to do are done safely in the way intended?

## Safety features

The labels illustrated in below show that equipment meets safety standards.

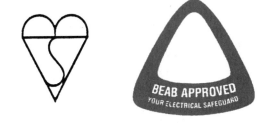

## Risk assessment

### How to identify safety hazards in the workplace

Employers have a legal responsibility to identify how much risk is involved in all the things that are done in the workplace. This is called risk assessment. The risk assessment helps to identify hazards (see below) before a new piece of equipment or working practice is introduced. A risk assessment is a careful examination of what could harm employees, visitors or clients in the workplace. The employer examines the situation and decides on what precautions are necessary to prevent harm to people. If this is done properly, no one should fall ill or be injured, nor cause injury to anyone else.

It is important to discover what causes accidents. The main way for an employer to prevent accidents is to first identify a hazard.

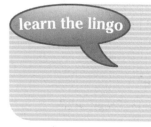

**learn the lingo**

A **hazard** is anything that can cause harm, including ill health and injury.

The **risk** is the chance, however high or low, that you, a service user or a visitor may be harmed by the hazard.

A hazard is anything that can cause harm, including ill health and injury. This can mean a wide range of things, from something that makes you cough to something that can kill you. Some substances can harm you in several different ways, e.g. you might breathe them in, swallow them or get them on your skin.

The risk is the chance, however high or low, that you, a service user or visitor may be harmed by the hazard.

### Carrying out a risk assessment

The questions an employer might ask when carrying out a risk assessment cover the following areas.

Tidiness

Are all parts of the premises clear of waste and rubbish, particularly:

- Storerooms?
- Attics and basements?
- Boiler rooms and other equipment rooms?
- Bottoms of lift shafts?
- Staircases and under the stairs?

Smoking

- Are enough ashtrays provided in all the areas where smoking is permitted?
- Are staff advised to use the ashtrays and not to throw cigarettes or matches into wastepaper bins, through gratings or out of windows?

Electricity

- Do all parts of the electrical installation comply with the Institution of Electrical Engineers (IEE) regulations for electrical installations?
- Is the electrical installation inspected and tested at least once every 5 years?
- Are staff trained to report frayed leads and faulty equipment?

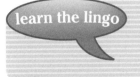

learn the lingo A **risk assessment** is a careful examination of what, in your workplace, could harm you, visitors or service users.

Heating appliances

- Are heating appliances fixed rather than portable?
- Do all heating appliances have adequate and secure fireguards?
- Are the staff warned to keep combustible materials away from heater?

Risk assessment needs to cover the following areas thoroughly:

- Fire
- First Aid and medication
- Child protection
- Staff safety measures
- Hygiene and tidiness
- Activities
- Outings and visits

- Electricity
- Heating and lighting
- Food and drink
- Security
- Internal features
- External features
- Storage.

## Fire

The effects of fire in the workplace can be very serious. Many people are killed each year by fire, and millions of pounds' worth of damage is caused.

### What can cause fire?

- Sparks from faulty electrical appliances and open fires
- Smoking materials such as matches, cigarette ends or pipe ash
- Cooker hobs
- Heating appliances such as fires and gas heaters.

### What should you do if you discover a fire?

You should notify a senior member of staff, who should:

- Ensure that the fire service has been called
- Go to the scene of the fire and supervise the fire fighting until the fire service arrives
- Clear everyone, except those actually engaged in fire fighting, from the immediate vicinity of the fire
- Order the evacuation of the building as soon as it becomes apparent that fire or smoke is spreading (before the fire is out of control)
- Take a roll call of all staff and residents or service users when the

premises have been evacuated (a list of absentees from the building should be available)

● Ensure that no one uses lifts.

Instructions should be given to caretakers and maintenance staff setting out the action they should take in the event of fire. This should include:

● Bringing all lifts to ground level and stopping them

● Shutting down all services not essential to the escape of occupants or likely to be required by the fire brigade

● Leaving lighting on.

You should know:

● The workplace evacuation procedures

● Where the activation points for the fire alarm are

● Where the fire extinguishers are

● What types of fire extinguisher are sited where

● How to operate the fire extinguishers.

On discovering fire, break the glass to activate the fire alarm or call someone. Close all windows and doors.

On hearing the fire alarm, close all doors and follow the evacuation procedure.

*A fire action notice*

---

### LITTLE TOTS NURSERY

#### FIRE RULES

If you discover a fire:
● Raise the alarm by operating the nearest fire alarm and proceed to the assembly point at the nearest exit (outside the Rest Room Exit)
● Go along the corridor through the Rest Room and out of the double-opening patio doors
● Close the door of your room as you leave and any others you may use
● Do not shout or run
● Study this notice carefully so that you will know what to do in an emergency
● Do not re-enter the building until told to do so by an appropriate person.

---

## Fire fighting

All workplaces must be inspected regularly by a fire officer to ensure that:

● Portable fire extinguishers and/or hose reels are provided in clearly visible and readily accessible places throughout the premises

● They are maintained at regular intervals

*All fire extinguishers should be maintained at regular intervals*

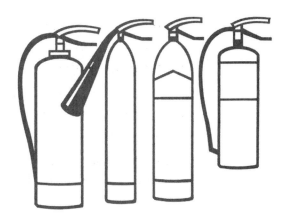

- Staff are familiar with their use
- Fire exits are clear and available for use.

Remember that you should only attempt to tackle small fires yourself with an extinguisher. If in doubt, call the fire service.

## Legislation

The government has passed laws to ensure that employers make the workplace safer. One of the most important laws is the Health and Safety at Work Act 1974.

*What is wrong in this picture?*

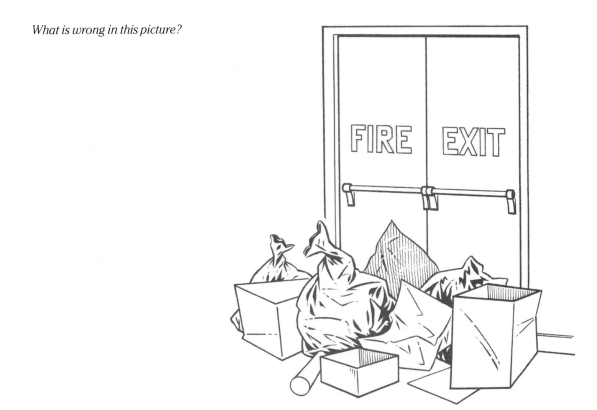

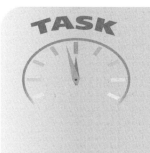

**TASK**

### Fire precautions

Draw a plan of your college, school or workplace. Look for all the different fire extinguishers and water hoses in public places and mark them on the plan.

Make notes of what kinds of fire the extinguishers are for.

Find out what the fire evacuation procedure is in your school, college or workplace. Explain this procedure clearly to your colleagues.

### Health and Safety at Work Act 1974

This is the law that controls health and safety in the workplace. Both employers and employees (you) have responsibilities under this law to protect the health and safety of yourselves and other people.

#### Responsibilities of the employer

An employer must provide a workplace that is safe from hazards and does not harm an employee's health. This includes:

- Having a safety policy
- Hygiene and welfare
- Comfort
- Cleanliness.

#### Safety policy

Employers must tell their staff how they are going to ensure their health and safety. This is called a safety policy. It should tell you:

- Who your key managers are, so that you can report any unsafe situation
- How they intend to protect you at work, including rules for safe procedures when carrying out particular tasks.

The safe procedure rules will cover, for example:

- The control of infection
- The wearing of protective clothing
- Using correct lifting procedures
- Training in the use of equipment.

The safety policy will, in many cases, be in the form of a booklet, or it may perhaps be a notice on a notice board. The document should also be published in a number of languages to make it accessible to all staff.

A manager of a residential home for elderly people, for example, or of a day centre for children must ensure that all staff know their duties so that

---

**Important rules**

- Learn how to work safely
- Obey safety rules
- Ask your supervisor or tutor if you don't understand any instruction or rule
- Report to your supervisor, manager or tutor anything that seems dangerous, damaged or faulty.

---

they pay appropriate attention to health and safety when they carry out their work. The maintenance of a safe environment and the practice of safe procedures enables the service user to feel secure and confident. That is one of the necessities of good social care. Make sure you know the safety rules and obey them.

## Hygiene and welfare

This includes:

- Separate marked toilets for each sex
- Toilets kept clean and in working order and ventilated
- Wash basin with hot and cold running water
- Soap, dryers and nail-brushes where appropriate
- Waste bins, regularly emptied
- Facilities for taking food and drink
- Safe methods for handling, storing and transporting materials. For example, drugs must be stored and used in such a way as to minimise risk to health. If a new cleaning product is introduced, an employer is obliged to tell employees of any possible harmful effects.

### Comfort

The employer should consider the comfort of employees, including:

- Making sure furniture is placed so that sharp corners do not present a danger to staff or service users

- Providing good ventilation in bathrooms, toilets, bedrooms

- Providing a thermometer in each work room so that staff can check temperature – this is important in areas where babies and young children are cared for

- Installing good lighting – particularly necessary when working with babies and young children.

### Cleanliness

The employer should ensure that:

- Workplace, furniture and fittings are kept clean

- All rubbish and waste food are regularly removed
- All spillages are cleaned up immediately
- Dirty linen is stored appropriately
- Dressings and medicines are disposed of according to instructions.

| PROHIBITION | MANDATORY | SAFE CONDITION | WARNING |
|---|---|---|---|
| Don't do | Must do | The safe way | Risk of danger |
| (red circle and red cross bar, for example 'No Smoking') | (blue circle, for example 'Wash your hands') | (green rectangle, for example 'First aid room') | (yellow triangle with black outline, for example 'Risk of electric shock') |

## Responsibilities of the employee

What are your responsibilities in the workplace as an employee? You have a duty to take reasonable care to avoid:

- Injury to yourself – for example, a nurse or care assistant who injures their back by not using the correct lifting procedures, when they were aware of them, would probably not be successful in claiming any compensation for their injury
- Injury to others – for example, if you injure a service user by not using the correct lifting procedure (after you have been trained) or by not using lifting aids, you may be liable to prosecution (that is, you may be taken to court). You must report any hazards or accidents to your employers.

---

It is your duty:
- To take care of yourself and anyone else – that means the children, their families and anyone who may be affected by your working activities
- To co-operate with your employer, helping in any way that you can to carry out the employer's duties under the Health and Safety at Work Act
- Not to tamper with or misuse anything provided by the employer.

---

For example, it would be the duty of a care worker looking after people in their own homes to take care of themselves and anyone else, the clients, their families and friends. The care worker has a responsibility not to tamper with or use any equipment, such as washing machines, irons, electric kettles or gas fires, that they feel is faulty or might cause harm to anyone.

As a care worker you should be prepared:

- By being dressed appropriately for work. Wear any protective clothing you have been given by your employer, such as overalls or rubber gloves. Also remember to wear well-fitting, comfortable shoes
- Always be on the look-out for safety hazards
- Report any hazards or accidents to your supervisor immediately
- Use only safe methods of working.

If you have any questions or worries about safety, talk to your tutor or supervisor in the workplace.

## What should you do if you are injured at work?

If you are injured at work:

- Report the accident to your immediate supervisor or tutor
- Record it in writing (it is usually recorded in an accident book)
- See a doctor – a medical examination should be carried after the accident and the result recorded.

## Safe procedures of work

Systems of work can affect your health and the client's health. For example, do you know what would happen to your work clothes if you were splashed by a chemical you were using to clean a floor? Could poor design of working areas like bathrooms lead to backache?

Are you aware of any potential safety hazard? Is there any risk of clients or patients transmitting disease? If you were working with old, unchecked electrical appliances in a client's home, would you know of the dangers or to whom to report your concerns? Are all students and staff aware of the procedures for staff who are vulnerable to physical violence?

### Control of Substances Hazardous to Health Regulations 1988 (COSHH)

A full description of COSHH is given in Unit 4, AO6.

### RIDDOR (Reporting of Injuries, Diseases and Dangerous Occurrences Regulations 1985)

Failure to comply with RIDDOR is a criminal offence. The Regulations require immediate notification by phone if anybody dies or is seriously injured in an accident at work or if there is a dangerous occurrence.

A written report must be sent within 7 days to confirm the above, and:

- If anyone is off work for more than 3 days as a result of an accident at work
- To report occupational diseases suffered by workers

### Co-operative play (3 years)

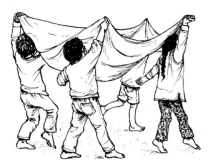

This is when children are beginning to play together and are willing to share. However there can still be disagreements.

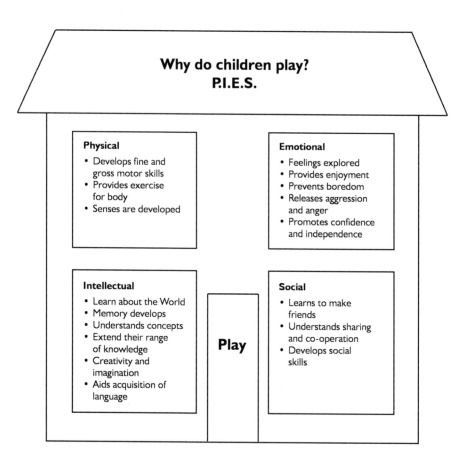

**Why do children play?**
**P.I.E.S.**

**Physical**
- Develops fine and gross motor skills
- Provides exercise for body
- Senses are developed

**Emotional**
- Feelings explored
- Provides enjoyment
- Prevents boredom
- Releases aggression and anger
- Promotes confidence and independence

**Intellectual**
- Learn about the World
- Memory develops
- Understands concepts
- Extend their range of knowledge
- Creativity and imagination
- Aids acquisition of language

**Play**

**Social**
- Learns to make friends
- Understands sharing and co-operation
- Develops social skills

## Types of play

There are several different types of play:

- Physical
- Creative
- Imaginative
- Manipulative
- Exploratory
- Social.

### Physical play

Physical play is to do with physical activities, for example riding a bike, climbing, swimming, or football. This is when children use their bodies in an active way, so it usually requires a lot of outdoor space. Physical activities promote fine and gross motor skill development, as well as improving balance and co-ordination. Physical play can involve children playing together, which encourages language development and social interaction. Emotionally, it helps to build self confidence.

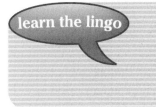

**learn the lingo**

**Gross motor skills** use the large muscles in the body and include activities such as running and cycling. **Fine motor skills** use the hands and fingers in precise actions such as writing, drawing, fastening shoelaces and buttons.

### Creative play

Creative play is when children use their imagination and their own ideas to make something that is original, such as a painting. It is easier for children to convey their thoughts and feelings through drawing and painting than through using their language skills, which may not yet be fully developed. Social skills can be developed when children are working on a group project, such as a collage. Hand–eye co-ordination and sensory skills are also developed.

### Imaginative play

This is pretend or role play and is part of a child's learning process. The child imagines that s/he is someone else, and acts out that role e.g. teacher, nurse, mother or father. As children interact with other children their social skills are enhanced. Expressing themselves in role play is another way of furthering their emotional development.

### Manipulative play

This is concerned with the skilful use of the hands. During this type of play the hands, eyes and brain have to work together. It includes activities such as playing with a rattle, building blocks, Lego, jigsaws, or playing with sand and water.

### Exploratory play

This allows a child to find out about the world around them by using all their senses. Initially, babies explore by placing objects in their mouths. This is known as *mouthing*. Older children use sensory exploration in a more meaningful way, and in this way concepts such as size, shape, weight, volume, texture and colour become understandable.

### Social play

Playing with others is a social activity. Children learn to share, to take turns and to co-operate with others. They learn what is socially acceptable behaviour.

## Design a suitable layout for a care and education setting for young children

*Floor plan of Bodgit's Nursery*

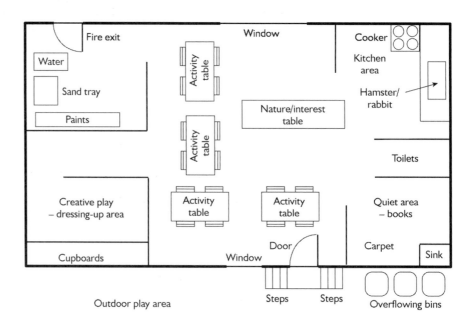

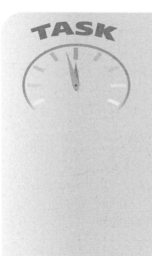

### Bodgit's Nursery

You are working as a nursery nurse at Bodgit's nursery. Assess the layout under the following headings:

Ergonomics; Safety; Access; Fit for Purpose; Safety Features.

Consider the following points when you are making your assessment:

- Is there access for people with disabilities?
- Are fire and other access points kept clear?
- Are activities that need water near to the sink?
- Is there enough space to allow children to move safely from one activity to another?

◄

- Is storage space located in areas accessible to all?
- Look at the four activity zones. Is there enough space for these activities? Are they located in the right areas? Do they all have the facilities they need?
- Is it a good idea to have the sink in the quiet area? If not, why not?
- Should the water, sand and painting activities be located together?
- Should a fire exit lead on to a major road? How could this be improved?
- Could the steps at the rear of the building be a problem?
- Should the hamster and rabbit be housed on the bench in the staff kitchen area?
- Should the kitchen area be open to children in the nursery?
- Should the toilets be near the kitchen area?
- Is there a hygiene issue with the bins?

## Different activities

- **Physical**

  Team games, e.g. rounders, cricket, football, netball, tennis

  Riding tricycle/bicycle, swings and playgroup equipment

  Hopscotch, tag or chasing

  Swimming

- **Creative**

  Painting and drawing

  Sand and water play

  Puppet shows

  Playdough, Plasticine

  Lego, bricks, collage

- **Structures**

  Bouncy castle, adventure playground, Wendy house

- **Discovery**

  Sand and water, different-sized beakers and containers, playdough, cooking, feeling different materials

- **Intellectual**

  Reading, computers, writing.

**AO6** **Plan and carry out an activity to intellectually stimulate young children and evaluate the success of the activity**

To help you decide what activity to chose you should have a long discussion with your teacher. Remember that the child's wishes and needs come first and that any thing you do must not disempower them or their carers or parents.

### Drawing up a plan

Planning is an important part of carrying out any task, activity or plan. When you have selected the child or children and identified the activity which will intellectually stimulate them, you will need to consider how long you have been given to carry out the plan.

The plan must include:

- The aims of the care
- Objectives of the plan
- Resources needed
- Timescales
- Cost.

### Objective of the plan – needs of the young child or children

- You must consider the physical, intellectual, emotional and social needs of the children involved.
- The health and safety issues relating to you, the children, equipment you might use and any material you might use.

### Timescales

- How long have you to carry out the activity?
- How available are any resources – the things you might need (jigsaws, board games, quizzes, Lego, paint, collage)
- Can you and child or children do all you want to do in the time given?
- Do you have the individual skills to complete the activity (organisational skills, interpersonal skills, communication skills, story telling skills, etc.)?

How do you evaluate the effectiveness of the activity?

## How to review the activity

When you have completed the activity, you will need to review your own individual performance against the tasks that you agreed to undertake with the child or children. To review the activity you will first need to look at whether you carried out the agreed activity.

You should look at:

- Own performance
- Did you achieve the original aim of the activity?
- Did you achieve the original objectives of the activity?
- How did you use the resources available?
- What were the outcomes of the activity?

### Review of your performance

To do this, you will need to look back at your original activity plan.

When reviewing what you have done, it often a very good idea to ask the people you did the activity with, the children, what they thought about it.

### Heath and safety considerations

When working in the health and social care services, we must always make sure that what we do does not make it hazardous for either the service user or ourselves. You must, therefore, take into consideration any health and safety factors of the activities you are planning.

## Assessment

a) You must individually

- Plan (the aim of the activity, objectives, resources, timescale)
- Set the criteria for measuring the success of the activity
- Carry out the activity
- Monitor (intellectual stimulation, safety) and
- Review the selected task.

b) You will need to consider the

- Physical, intellectual, emotional and social needs of the children/ child
- Intellectual stimulation of the children/child
- Health and safety issues.

c) It is very important that you consider how you can involve the children in planning the activity so as to empower them.

d) When you have carried out the chosen activity you must assess your own performance.

- Did you achieve the aims that you set yourself?
- Did you achieve the objectives of the activity?
- Did you make the best use of available resources?

– Did you meet the outcomes that you set for yourself?

– Look at your own strengths – what did you do best?

– What could you have done better?

– How did you empower the children/child?

– What improvements would you make in future?

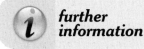

**further information**

Clarke L (2000) *Health and Social Care for Foundation GNVQ.* Nelson Thornes, Cheltenham

Clarke L (2000) *Health and Social Care for Intermediate GNVQ.* Nelson Thornes, Cheltenham

Clarke L (2002) *Health and Social Care GCSE.* Nelson Thornes, Cheltenham

Dare A and O' Donovan M (2003) *A Practical Guide to Working with Babies* 3rd edn. Nelson Thornes, Cheltenham

Minett P (1994) *Child Care and Development.* John Murray, London

Tassoni P (2000) *Certificate in Child Care and Education,* 2nd edn Heinemann, Oxford

www.cache.org.uk – Cache

www.capt.org.uk – Child Safety

www.childcarelink.gov.uk – CHILD Care link

www.dfes.gov.uk/childcare – Department of Education and Skills

www.early-years-nto.org.uk – Early Years Training

www.ofsted.gov.uk – OFSTED

www.pat.org.uk – Professional Association of Nursery Nurses

www.socialworkcareers.co.uk – Social Work Careers

## Summary

- Young children can be looked after in a wide variety of settings, including private day nurseries, workplace crèches and local authority nurseries.

- Young children can be looked after by a variety of carers, each having slightly different roles and demanding different levels of qualification, but the same skills and qualities. They include nursery nurses, playgroup leaders and childminders.

- A risk assessment should be carried out in the workplace and safety hazards must be identified and removed. Any accidents must be reported to a line manager and/or written down in an accident book if one is used.

- Children play in a variety of ways for a variety of reasons, which are broadly physical, intellectual, emotional and social.

- The layout of a nursery should be assessed for ergonomics, safety, access and being fit for purpose.

# Preparing to work with older service users

**9**

## To complete this unit you will need to:

- Describe the different types of provision for older service users and their purpose
- Recognise particular needs of older service users
- Promote and maintain a safe environment for older service users
- Demonstrate effective communication when responding to requests for support from older service users and assess own performance
- Carry out practical tasks for older service users and assess own performance
- Carry out a recreational activity with older service users and assess own performance.

**AO1** Describe the different types of provision for older service users and their purpose

### Introduction

When discussing services for older people we are usually referring to people who are past retirement age. In men this is at 65 years and for women there is the option of retiring at 60, otherwise it is also 65 years.

Old age is not necessarily a time of problems. Many older people will not require assistance from carers. There is no standard model older person. Older people differ widely in needs, lifestyles and expectations. Also, they have the same emotional and human needs as young people.

While age cannot be equated automatically with dependency, many people, as they grow older, find themselves generally slowing down. Some of their faculties (eyesight, hearing, speech, etc.) may start to decline or certain disabilities may develop.

The ageing body is increasingly subject to degenerative diseases. These are diseases that gradually worsen over time and can be any of the following:

- Atheroma – a gradual build-up of fatty deposits on the walls of the arteries giving rise to coronary heart disease and strokes
- Osteoarthritis – where changes occur in the joints, giving rise to pain and loss of mobility
- Brain degeneration – caused by either Alzheimer's disease, in which the nerve cells of the brain degenerate excessively, or atheroma of the arteries supplying the brain; both these conditions can lead to gradual loss of intellectual power and ability
- Cancer – there is an increase in the incidence of many cancers with advancing age.

## Provision for older service users

Many services used by children, adolescents and adult people are also available to support the older person – primary health services, health promotion, hospital services and residential care. However some services are specific to the needs of older service users.

It must be remembered that, although older people have poorer health than younger people, ageing does not cause disease. Older people with better health habits keep healthier for longer. Regular physical activity can increase how long an older person lives. For most older people the benefits of activity outweigh the risks.

Remember that the majority of older people require no care or care only occasionally.

The decline of the family unit means that fewer older people are being looked after by relatives and this puts increased pressure upon day care and domiciliary services.

## Day care

Day centres and residential homes provide a variety of services. For example, they provide a place where people meet socially, offering opportunities for conversation and other forms of social recreation.

They also provide intellectual activity in a variety of ways.

- They often offer the opportunity to play games, both group games, such as bingo, and individual challenges, such as chess and draughts.
- For some people, intellectual stimulation has to be organised on a one-to-one basis by the care workers. Conversation with care workers, involving remembering things that have happened in the past, is important. Using photographs and things from the past to stimulate

*Services for older service users*

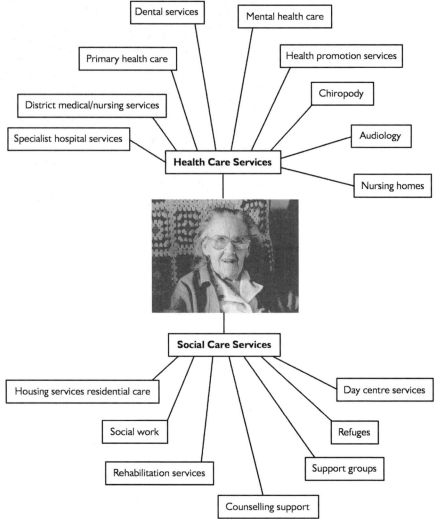

memories also enables people to think about the present.

- Intellectual recreation can also include activities related to occupational therapy. Intellectual activity may come from concentrating on painting, sewing or knitting. It may come from practising a skill like cooking. All of these also provide a degree of physical activity. They do not provide exercise like swimming, but they require fine movements and help maintain hand and finger mobility.

## Residential provision

Residential care includes a number of services that are provided for people who have left their own homes for whatever reason.

Residential care differs from care in a person's own home in that, when in residential care, users receive special organised care in which the needs of other residents have to be balanced against their own. In residential care people may have to go to bed at a specific time because of lack of staff, or

*Day care for older service users*

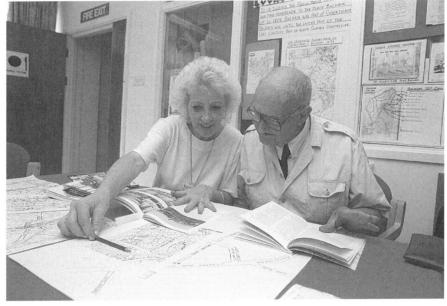

take their meals at certain times. They may not have choice over meals or who their GP is.

However they will have security, companionship, and have their basic needs of food, shelter and warmth met. The kind of care that each residential care facility offers depends on the needs of the residents who live there.

## Sheltered housing

Sheltered housing fulfils a housing need – it meets the special needs of many older people. Sheltered housing also reduces the possibility of emergencies occurring, through the presence of a warden. This type of housing offers more choice to older people, as it is an alternative to residential care. Sheltered housing also help to combat loneliness by offering the possibility of wider social contacts, and it fosters independence.

Sheltered housing usually has:

- A resident warden
- An alarm system fitted to each dwelling
- Occupancy restricted to older people only
- Accommodation all on one site
- In many cases a common room and common dining area for those who wish to take their meals there.

There are, however, various degrees of 'shelter' based upon the amount of communal facilities provided.

## Hospice care

Hospice care began in the UK in the 1960s. The modern hospice movement now offers active total care, called palliative care, to dying people whose disease no longer responds to drugs or medical care. This approach allows people who are dying to live with dignity until their death.

The hospice offers care in a number of ways by offering short- or long-term care and pain management. The care offered attempts to see the person as a whole with social, emotional, psychological and medical needs.

## Personal care

Domiciliary care is offered to older people living in their own homes. People receive these services – home carer or meals-on-wheels – when recovering from illness or in the long term because they are unable to manage on their own. Older service users who are frail and dependent may wish to stay in their own homes rather than enter residential care.

Older people benefit from living in their own homes – they are near friends and relatives and can go to bed or eat a meal whenever they like. They are allowed to make decision for themselves: this is known as empowerment.

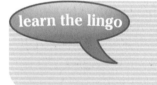
**learn the lingo**

**Empowerment** means giving people the opportunity to make their own choices about their lives.

However, there may be some disadvantages to living at home when older people are dependent on others. Care staff may not be available to get them up out of bed in the morning or help them to go to bed at times they wish. Friends may not be living near and relatives may have died or live far away.

*A home carer can help older service users stay in their own home*

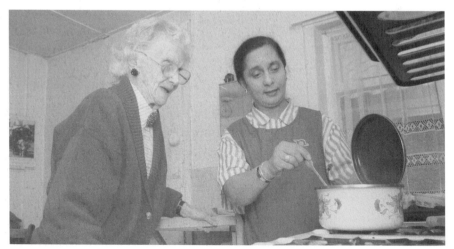

### Home care

A number of home care staff provide emotional, social and practical support to older service users living in their own homes in the community. Local authorities have a duty (this means they must do it) to provide home helps (now officially called home care assistants or home carers). Many home care assistants work for private organisations and offer people a service in their own homes for a fee.

Home care assistants carry out tasks such as simple cleaning, lighting fires, shopping, cooking and basic personal tasks. They also write letters and provide social support. Most of their work is concerned with supporting older service users but they do also work with people with physical disabilities and families with young children.

### Meals-on-wheels provision

This service is becoming increasingly important as more and more older dependent people choose to live in their own homes. About 33 million meals are provided every year in England to people in their own homes. This service is provided by the local authority in many areas but it is still also offered by voluntary agencies such as the Women's Royal Voluntary Service, or the Women's Institute in rural areas.

Meals-on-wheels services are among the most important forms of community support for older service users in their own homes. Meals-on-wheels makes a contribution to their nutritional needs and is often the only social contact that they have during the week. The service can also improve the morale of older people. As older service users are most susceptible to hypothermia and falls, the daily visit of meals-on-wheels staff can provide a check that all is well.

*Meals-on-wheels*

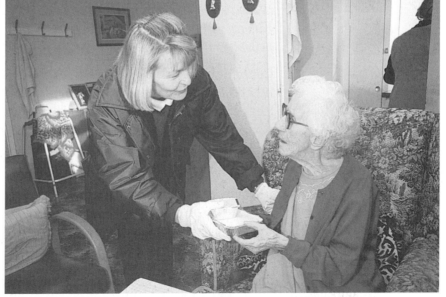

## Health provision

The care provided by the NHS means that anyone in the UK can visit their general practitioner (GP) whenever they feel ill, without having to pay anything. The role of the doctor is to:

- Diagnose – find out what is wrong with the patient
- Prescribe – decide on the treatment to help the patient
- Monitor – review the condition of the patient and change the treatment if necessary.

Most nurses are to be found working in hospitals alongside hospital doctors. There are two levels of personnel in the nursing team currently employed in the NHS: registered general nurses (RGNs) and health care assistants (HCAs), who support the RGNs.

### General practitioner provision

General practitioners form part of the front line of the NHS and work in that part of the service called 'primary care'. Services offered by GPs are generally free to patients, although there are flat rate charges for some services to some patients. Children, older people and those on low incomes get their prescriptions free.

### Nursing provision in the community

Health authorities have a responsibility to provide nurses to assist with treatment in a patient's home. **Community nurses** (formerly **district nurses**) provide support and nursing care for acute and chronic patients of all ages, but predominantly for older people in their own homes. They also provide the link between hospitals and the primary health care team by referring their patients to other carers and services.

The role of the **health visitor** is in the area of health education, prevention of illness and promotion of health in antenatal classes and health clinics, monitoring the development of children and working with patients in their own homes. The health visitor also has a large part to play in the community care of older people.

**Community psychiatric nurses** (CPNs) and the community-based **mental handicap nurses** (RNMHs) provide continuing care and support for people who have been receiving hospital care, perhaps long-term, and who are now returning to life in the community. The link between health and social care for these patients is through social workers and community-based nurses.

**Physiotherapists** have an important role in improving the mobility of older service users, using supportive and manipulative exercises to develop muscles for movement. Physiotherapists improve the health and function of service users through simple corrective exercises. They often use equipment such as infrared and ultrasound machines. They work in co-operation with doctors to plan physiotherapy programmes.

**Occupational therapists** (OTs) work in the NHS to treat illness, both mental and physical, through activity. They work on a one-to-one basis, with groups and with recreational activities. The aim is to rehabilitate service users and teach them basic living skills. Many OTs work in the community and are also employed by Social Services Departments, offering advice on aids and adaptations for daily living.

**Case Study**

Maria is a confused old lady. She has lived alone for many years since her husband died. She lives in a large house and managed to cope on her own until she fell and damaged her hip. Since her fall she has become more and more confused and, as a result, sometime does not recognise the postman or the milkman. She also sometimes leaves the gas on without lighting it. An occupational therapist has recommended aids and adaptations to her home and a physiotherapist comes in to help her exercise her leg.

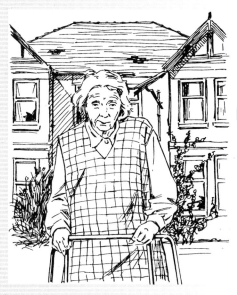

Maria has no relatives. She has difficulty getting her pension every week. She is now so frail that she can no longer cook her own meals and because of her hip injury cannot get in or out of bed without the help of a home carer.

*Would you break confidentially in any of these situations? If you think you would, why?*

*What has happened to Maria? Explain*

*Describe the role of each professional caring for Maria*

*What do you think will happen to Maria now?*

*The care team that will help and support Maria*

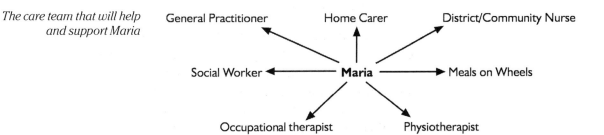

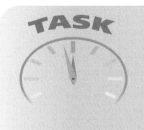

**Different types of provision for older service users and their purpose**

Identify in your local community as many services that support elderly people as you can. The location of these can be identified on a map of the area.

You should also describe the differences between the types of provision you have identified such as the differences between personal care and support, nursing care, help to live independently and care of the dying.

## Recognise particular needs of older service users

One of the ways we build relationships with older service users is by showing them that we have up-to-date knowledge about the services that are available and how these services can help them.

Before you can give any advice, however, you need to find out what a service user's needs are. How do you do this? First you have to carry out an assessment of the service user's situation – their abilities, expectations and aspirations. You do this by looking at the service user's needs under the following headings:

- Physical needs
- Emotional needs
- Intellectual needs
- Social and cultural needs.

### How are a service user's needs recognised?

#### *Maslow's theory of human needs*

This theory is a useful starting point. Maslow suggests that human needs are arranged in a series of five levels as shown on page 283.

The needs at level 1, such as shelter, food and water, are the basic, essential requirements for any individual to live. The more complex needs shown from the middle of the pyramid upwards are only considered when the basic needs have been taken care of. For example, a homeless, hungry person needs shelter and food before beginning to worry about their social needs.

- **Level 1: Basic physical needs** – These include the need to satisfy hunger and thirst, the need for oxygen and the need to keep warm or cool. These also include the need for sleep, sensory pleasures, maternal behaviour and sexual desire. If people are denied any of these needs,

*Maslow's hierarchy of needs*

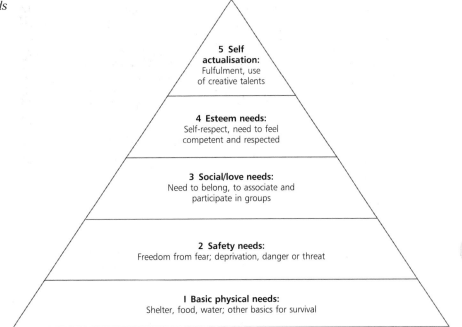

they may spend long periods of time looking for them. For example, if water or food is not readily available, most people's energies will be spent trying to obtain a supply.

- **Level 2: Safety needs** – Once basic physical needs have been met, a person's next concern is usually for safety and security, freedom from pain and from threat of physical attack, and protection from danger.

- **Level 3: Love and social needs** – These include affection, a sense of belonging, the need for social activities, friendships, and the giving and receiving of love.

- **Level 4: Self-esteem needs** – These include the need to have self-respect and to have the esteem of others. Self-respect involves the desire to have confidence, strength, independence, freedom and achievement. The esteem of others involves having prestige, status, recognition, attention, reputation and appreciation from other people.

- **Level 5: Self actualisation/self-fulfilment needs** – This is the development and realisation of your full potential. All the other needs in the pyramid have to be achieved before you can reach this stage.

Another way to define an older service user's needs is by using the 'activities of daily living' model, looking at the service user's situation in relation to the everyday activities that people need to carry out. These activities include:

- **Safe environment** – freedom from pain, comfort

- **Body functions** – breathing comfortably, passing urine and faeces regularly, maintaining body temperature, etc.

- **Nutrition** – a healthy diet, ability to eat, adequate and suitable fluids
- **Personal cleaning and dressing** – mouth, teeth, eyes, ears, skin, suitable clothing, ability to dress and undress
- **Mobility** – can the service user get out of bed or exercise?
- **Sleep** – sleep pattern, does the service user wake during the night or sleep during the day?
- **Sexuality** – is the service user able to express their feelings? Do they have the ability to enter into meaningful sexual relationships?
- **Religion** – are the cultural needs of service user being met? Do they have the freedom to worship as they wish?
- **Communication** – is the service user able to communicate verbally, express emotions, use smell, touch?

## Physical needs

These may be met by:

- The provision of appropriate food and drink – for example, babies and people who are ill (such as someone suffering from diabetes) need different diets from healthy older people
- Attending to personal hygiene – this is essential to prevent infection and the spread of disease.

### Physical illness or conditions

Some of the physical changes that are happening throughout life and that may become more obvious in old age are listed below.

- **Skin** – dryness, wrinkling and loss of elasticity occur.
- **Hair** – growth slows, thinning occurs, men may go bald and all hair goes grey.
- **Eyesight** – the ability to focus close up disappears. People find it harder to distinguish colours. Going from brightly lit places into the dark becomes a problem. Side vision becomes more narrow. The medical conditions cataracts and glaucoma can lead to blindness if left untreated.
- **Hearing** – the ability to hear deteriorates. Appreciation of high-pitch frequencies is lost first.
- **Smell and taste** – these senses deteriorate, sometimes causing loss of appetite.
- **Teeth** – may deteriorate quite early in life. Gum disease and decay are major problems. Carers need to be sensitive to this when providing food and attending to oral hygiene.
- **The lungs and respiratory system** – the lungs become less elastic and respiratory muscles weaken. Older people are more likely to be affected by lung disorders.

- **The heart and blood vessels** – the efficiency of the heart decreases. Blood vessels become less elastic and blood pressure may be raised.
- **The digestive system** – secretions of saliva and digestive juices decrease with age. Food takes much longer to pass through the body as muscles become weaker and less effective. Constipation can then become a problem.
- **The urinary system** – the kidneys become less efficient at filtering out waste products effectively.
- **The reproductive system** – in women the menopause will have marked the end of reproductive life.
- **The skeleton and muscles** – between the ages of 20 and 70 a person can lose 5cm in height. Total bone mass is reduced and muscles become less flexible. Posture and mobility are likely to be altered considerably.

This all sounds negative. There is no denying that certain aspects of the ageing process can be very troublesome to some individuals, but not to everyone.

### Intellectual and emotional needs

These may be more difficult to meet. It is important to:

- Treat people as individuals
- Respect people's individuality and opinions
- Allow people to be as independent as possible.

For example, in a residential home for older people these needs may be met by allowing residents to:

- Be independent
- Choose their own meals
- Make decisions about their own meal times, bed times, visiting times, etc.
- Participate in social and educational activities within the establishment and outside it.

Emotional needs are not separate from physical needs. People often feel better after a bath or a visit to the hairdresser. If they feel clean, they feel more secure when interacting with others. For example, someone who smells of urine will not feel emotionally secure when talking to relatives or friends. By meeting their physical need, their emotional need may also be met.

Loss, disability or illness can occur at any age. However we are only now beginning to appreciate the effect of loss in old age. Many people remain remarkably fit into extreme old age and stay strong and mentally agile. However, there are many losses that affect the older person, including:

- Loss of status and defined role (such as worker, wife, mother)
- Loss of company, for example through the death of a partner, friends or pets
- Loss of income
- Loss of bodily function
- Loss of health
- Loss of sexual function
- Loss of independence and home following admission to residential care or hospital.

## Mental health needs of older service users

### Personality

It is often said that old people do not like change. Like most of us, older people find familiar surroundings and situations a comfort.

They are less likely to make mistakes in their own homes than when in hospital or residential care.

### Memory

You may notice that some older people easily forget what happened yesterday but remember clearly things that happened 50 years ago. This may be because of the way the memory works – earlier events are fixed in the brain by repetition (the person may have experienced a particular event a number of times). The brain remembers these earlier events rather than more recent events.

### Learning and intelligence

Older people do tend to take longer to absorb new information than younger people but they do not become less intelligent. Many older people take Open University degrees or enrol in classes in local colleges.

### Social aspects of ageing

The main social aspects of ageing are:

- Retirement
- Family changes
- Loneliness
- Changing role.

## Personal care and support for older service users

When their children have grown up, many older people will become grandparents and great-grandparents. Older people do have a considerable role to play in looking after their grandchildren, often providing vital child care and sometimes even giving financial help.

Drastic changes are brought about when one partner dies. The remaining partner may have little experience of managing financial matters. They may not drive or feel confident to attend functions by themselves or they may lack the ability to cook and care for themselves and their home.

People can be isolated in their own homes because of poor mobility or because they do not have many visitors or friends. It is also possible for people to feel extremely lonely when they live in residential homes. They may have difficulty in forming relationships with other residents and staff. Many people in residential care or hospital miss their own homes and familiar possessions.

Many older people worry that their declining health may cause them to be a burden to other people. An older person may become totally dependent on one of their children – the roles have been reversed.

### Social and cultural needs

These are an important aspect of a person's life. Social needs can be met by:

- Encouraging people to socialise
- Encouraging people to keep in touch with relatives and friends
- Arranging for volunteers to visit them in their own homes if they are housebound.

Cultural needs are recognised when people are allowed to practise their cultural rituals and traditions. They can be met by recognising that people:

- Need to be able to practise their religion
- May have cultural food preferences
- Relate to other members of the family differently in different cultures.

### Support for older services users

Older service users have the right to independence and privacy and should have opportunities to participate in the life of their local communities but these rights are very often not respected. This can be a particular problem when people are cared for in residential or day care.

Every person has access to health and social care services but many may not know of their rights because they cannot read or speak English.

Most health and social care organisations have published pamphlets and leaflets describing their services and how people can use them, for instance codes of practice or charters. These sources of information are often published in languages other than English, such as Chinese and Gujarati. Many hospitals have appointed workers, the Patient Advocacy Service, to act for patients and take up any complaints they may have.

They also provide interpreters to help service users whose first language is not English.

Many organisations are dedicated to supporting service users in receiving adequate services. Sources of help and support can also be obtained from the Citizen's Advice Bureau, local council advice officers and the local Community Health Council.

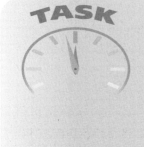

## The particular needs of older service users

Identify and describe the

1. Physical
2. Social and
3. Emotional

needs of older service users who

a. Have mental health needs
b. Have a physical illness or condition
c. Need personal care and support.

 **AO3** Promote and maintain a safe environment for older service users

### Protecting service users from harm

The **Heath and Safety at Work Act 1974** (HASAWA 1974) is the law that controls health and safety in the workplace. Employers (the person you work for) and employees (you) have responsibilities under this law to protect the health and safety of yourselves and other people.

### What responsibilities has the employer?

The employer must:

1. Make your workplace **safe** and **without any risk** to your health

   The employer should consider the comfort and safety of employees, including:

   – Making sure furniture is placed so that sharp corners do not present a danger to staff or service users

   – Providing good ventilation in bathrooms, toilets, bedrooms

   – Providing a thermometer in each work room so that staff can check temperature – this is important in areas where elderly people are cared for

- Installing good lighting – particularly necessary when working with babies and young children

- Making sure that there is adequate lighting and ventilation in all rooms.

2. Make sure that any **equipment** that you might use during your work is **safe to use**

The employer should ensure that:

- Workplace, furniture and fittings are kept clean

- All rubbish and waste food are regularly removed

- All spillages are cleaned up immediately

- Dirty linen is stored appropriately

- Dressings and medicines are disposed of according to instructions.

3. Give you **details** of how to **work safely** with any equipment that you may use

The employer **must** give you instructions or training before you use any machinery or equipment that is necessary to do your job. You may get manufacturers' instructions – manuals that tell you about the machine. You should never use machinery or equipment unless you are trained to do so.

4. Make sure that any **dangerous** equipment and substances (poisons, drugs, cleaning fluids for example) are moved, stored and used **safely**.

- For example, drugs must be stored and used in a way as to minimise risk to health.

- If you are asked to use a new cleaning product, the employer is obliged to tell you of any possible harmful effects that it may have.

5. Keep **dust, fumes and noise** under control

6. Let you have **access** to adequate **welfare facilities** (e.g. rest rooms, canteens)

The employer should:

- Provide separate marked toilets for each sex and keep them clean, in working order and ventilated

- Provide wash basins, hot and cold running water, soap, dryers and nail brushes where appropriate

- Provide a supply of wholesome drinking water

- Keep the place clean and make sure that waste bins are regularly emptied

- Provide facilities for taking food and drink.

### What is a safety policy?

Employers must tell their staff how they are going to make sure of their health and safety. This is called a safety policy. It should tell you:

- Who your managers are, so that you can report any unsafe things you find
- How your employer intends to protect you at work. This should cover, for example:
  - How to stop infections
  - The wearing of protective clothing
  - Using correct lifting procedures
  - Training in the use of equipment.

The safety policy will usually be in the form of a booklet, or it might perhaps be a notice on a notice board.

The safety policy should also be published in a number of languages to make it accessible to all staff.

Sometimes the employer will put up a poster published by the Health and Safety Executive called 'Health and Safety Law: What you should know'. Look for any posters displayed in your workplace and read what they say.

### Important rules

- Learn how to work safely
- Obey safety rules
- Ask your supervisor or tutor if you don't understand any instruction or rule
- Report to your supervisor, manager or tutor anything that seems dangerous, damaged or faulty

### What can you do about hazards in care settings?

Large organisations (such as factories, colleges and hospitals) usually have:

- A health and safety officer, who will have the overall responsibility for health and safety policy
- A system for reporting defects in equipment
- An accident book for recording accidents.

If you suspect that equipment is faulty do not use it. Report your suspicions as soon as possible.

### What are the responsibilities of the employee in the workplace?

What are your responsibilities in the workplace?

You have a right to have **clear safety instructions**. For example, do you know what would happen to your work clothes if you were splashed by a chemical you were using to clean a floor? Could poor design of working areas like bathrooms or service users beds or chairs lead to backache when you clean them?

You must be able to **work safely**, with the right equipment. For example, carers should have hoists for lifting people out of bed or into the bath. You should have the right equipment to do the job safely.

You should not be working long hours; lorry drivers are only allowed to drive for a certain length of time before they must stop and rest. If your employer makes you work long hours you may get tired and injure yourself or a service user. **People make mistakes when they are tired**.

Your employer will provide you with **protective clothing** when you do certain jobs, for example when working in a kitchen you should wear an overall and, if you come into contact with food, a cap that covers your hair. When handling dirty linen you should wear an overall and rubber gloves to protect yourself from infection.

### Safe working systems – a checklist

- Do you know who your supervisor is?
- Who do you report accidents and hazards to?
- Do you know the safe ways of doing the job?
- Are you are using equipment? Have you been instructed in its use and limitations?
- Has anyone assessed whether the equipment you are using is safe for the job?
- If things go wrong, do you know what to do?
- Are you aware of a system for checking that jobs you are asked to do are done safely in the way intended?

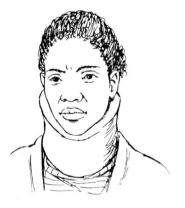

### Employees responsibility

In the last section we looked at many of your rights, now we will look at what responsibilities you have to keep the workplace as safe as possible.

## Factors that motivate people to communicate

### The physical environment

The physical environment is also a major factor in effective communication. Interaction needs to occur in an appropriate environment. If confidentiality is a concern, privacy will be important, so that the interaction will not be overheard. Too much noise or too many distractions can seriously inhibit the effectiveness of an interaction. Comfortable seating can also help.

### How the space in the care setting is actually laid out can affect communication.

How the space in the care setting is actually laid out affects service users' and care workers' behaviour in two ways. Physical restrictions may limit or direct the behaviour of people in the care setting as well as having psychological effects. Issues such as noisiness and privacy are important. Walls are good in that they may provide some privacy, but they may also create isolation. Both privacy and the opportunity for interaction are necessary, and creating the right balance in the physical environment is not easy. In all care services, space configuration is an important consideration where interviews or interaction will occur. In residential and day services, the location of lounges, eating areas, administrative facilities, bedrooms, activity areas and so on determine what relationships are formed, who people approach for help and advice, and who they trust.

### Heating, lighting etc.

This aspect of the physical setting includes lighting, heating, levels and types of noise, odours and general cleanliness. These rather subtle variables can have a significant influence on the degree of comfort the service user experiences. Making service users comfortable is important. The physical ambience in the office, for example, should communicate that visitors are welcome. Generally, people feel more comfortable in 'warm' environments where there are soft seats, subdued lighting, carpets, curtains and pot plants. By involving service users, and avoiding harsh furnishings and lighting, the care setting can be optimised for supporting interpersonal interaction.

## Main barriers to communication and poor relationships

Physical or practical factors, such as noise or interruptions, or barriers like desks or chairs, may spoil or stop good communication with the other person. Sometimes the room temperature may be so cold or so hot that it is difficult to concentrate on the matter in hand. You or the service user may be very tired or hungry. Children and many adults find it hard to take in what is being said if they are tired, thirsty or hungry.

As well as physical barriers affecting your rapport with the other person, there may be language problems or a speech difficulty, which will slow down the interaction.

### Lack of respect and not maintaining confidentiality

If you break confidentiality you are betraying trust and this will affect communication with the older service user. If someone trusts you sufficiently to talk to you deeply about themselves or their problems, then that trust should never be broken. It is demeaning to the other person if you chat about them openly. It would also be very distressing to anyone who knew the other person. If you need help yourself because of what a service user has told you, then you must go to the supervisor in private.

## Assess own performance

To develop your skills you will need to assess your own performance in terms of your strengths, your development needs, the benefits to the service user and the method that you used to empower the older person.

*Table 9.1  Assess your performance*

| Performance | Your strengths | Your weaknesses | Your development needs | Benefits to the service user |
| --- | --- | --- | --- | --- |
| Responding to needs of older service users | | | | |
| Communication skills | | | | |
| Understanding of factors that motivate people | | | | |
| Understanding of main barriers to communication | | | | |

## Empowerment

### Using effective communication to empower

Interaction between care workers and service users should be empowering for the service user. Class, age, disability, gender and race may all contribute to individuals feeling that they lack power – that they are somehow 'unequal' to others. One of the goals of effective interaction is to equalise relationships and to establish a sense of partnership with service users. Skilful listening and questioning, as explained below, can help to empower service users. Awareness of people's rights and preferences, helping people to talk about the past and listening attentively to service users' experiences can all help to empower. Of course, gaining consent from service users to explore issues with them is central to any interview or formal interaction.

### Why is it important to empower service users?

Effective communication in health and care services can only ever be empowering because:

- it respects people's preferences and beliefs

Table 9.2  Assessment of methods used to empower older service users

| Performance | Your strengths | Your weaknesses | Your development needs | Benefits to the service user |
|---|---|---|---|---|
| Respect for the older person's preferences and beliefs | | | | |
| Promoting confidentiality | | | | |
| Allowing older people to express their views | | | | |
| Promoting older people's rights | | | | |
| Develop the older person's individual identity | | | | |
| Supporting the older person's personal development | | | | |

- it promotes confidentiality and respects people's privacy
- it enables service users to express their views and be heard
- it promotes service users' rights
- it helps to develop individual identities in service users and supports personal development.

There are many people involved in providing services and assistance to an older service user. All these carers must work together to provide the best service possible. It is also important that they co-operate very closely with the relatives and friends of the service user.

However, most important of all is that everyone, professional workers and informal carers, must take into account, and act upon, the wishes of the service user. What the service user wants is the most important thing, not what is available to offer them or what we as carers might think is the best thing for them. It is the older person who must have the final say in what services and support they want.

So that the service user can make informed decisions, the carer should:

- Explain what process they are involved in
- Let the service user put forward their own views
- Agree with the service user what services they would wish
- Talk through with the service user how the services can be delivered
- Involve the service user fully in reviewing the situation as appropriate.

The voluntary organisations play an important role in the provision of care for older dependent people. They can be very flexible in the services they provide and how they provide them. They are not bound by rules and regulations, which may hinder statutory services. (See Unit 1 to remind yourself about statutory organisations.)

Voluntary organisations and self-help groups can be of great help to older people, particularly those who are housebound. They can:

- Provide information about services available and help people get appropriate support
- Provide information about assistive equipment
- Visit and provide support – Age Concern, for example, provides a wide range of services for older people:

    - Visiting service for older people, offering companionship
    - Good neighbour scheme, provision of visiting, shopping, gardening and other household tasks
    - Holidays
    - Telephone link – volunteers contact the housebound older person at pre-arranged time each day to check they are OK and also to offer support

- Day centres
- Coffee shops and luncheon clubs
- Free transport.

### Who gives care?

Other groups, such as the Association of Stroke Clubs, provide self-help and information to members. Crossroads is a voluntary scheme providing a support system for people in their own homes by offering temporary or regular care relief. This provides support and a rest for the carer by allowing the volunteer to attend to the personal needs of the service user.

Six million people are involved in providing voluntary services in the UK. The day-to-day work that the volunteers do is varied. They offer an informal system of caring that bridges the gap between the older service user and the statutory services.

## How can service users be empowered and why is it important?

One of the ways in which we can help service users to maintain their dignity and independence is to give them choice and allow them to make decisions that affect their lives.

Giving this choice is central to the quality of care. It takes the power and control from the carer and places it where it belongs, with the service user. Society, that is us, tends not to listen to people who have disabilities. However, by offering choice to people we empower them. This gives them a sense of dignity and worth.

We can empower older people by:

- Being sensitive to their needs
- Listening to what they are saying
- Not 'talking down' to them
- Not labelling those people with disabilities
- Negotiating with the service user, carer and any other professionals
- Giving appropriate support as necessary.

Older people should be encouraged to make their own decisions and to be involved as much as possible in making decisions about their own lives. In this way we empower people and allow them to keep their dignity and self-respect.

Did your answer to the questions in the case study about Jack Glen include any of the following?

- Ask Jack what he wanted
- Explain to him what was available to help his mobility problem

Jack Glen was bereaved by the loss of his wife, upon whom he depended a great deal. A few weeks later he suffered a stroke, which restricted his mobility and physical competence: 'I felt helpless and lonely at home and I think I was getting depressed. I wanted to go into an old people's home, but the social worker and home help kept telling me that I was better off in my own home. I got very angry but was afraid to argue in case they wouldn't give me any help.'

*Do you think that the social worker and the home help were empowering Jack? How could they have made him feel better and worth listening to?*

- Ask him if he would mind being visited by an occupational therapist or physiotherapist
- Discuss with him the results of any assessment
- Let him make the final choice.

## AO5 Carry out practical tasks for older service users and assess own performance

### Serving a snack and drinks to a group of older people with disabilities

Refer to the section on care planning earlier in this chapter. Assess the needs of the service users to find out:

- How much they can do for themselves?
- Any special diets including cultural and religious factors?
- Likes, dislikes and choices.

Plan exactly what you are going to do. Prepare:

- Set the tables so that they look attractive – don't forget salt, pepper and sauces
- Set out specially adapted cutlery if required
- Have a jug of water or other drinks with glasses or special feeding cups
- A few small flowers look very nice
- Have napkins and possibly special bibs to protect clothing from food
- Make sure the seating arrangements are appropriate – perhaps some service users will come to the table in wheelchairs or may need to sit in a specially adapted chair. The height of the table and the space available must be considered.

Carry out the task:

- Make sure that everyone has had the opportunity to go to the lavatory and to wash their hands

- Make sure they are comfortably seated in a place where they like to sit
- Serve the food and drink, making sure that carers are available to assist service users who are not able to feed themselves.

About the food – food and drink should:

- Take into account the dietary needs, culture and religion of the service user
- Look appetising
- Smell good
- Taste good
- Be served at the right temperature
- Be in the right quantity for the particular service user.

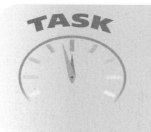

## Diet in different cultures

Find out about a diet from a different culture.

Write up your findings.

### Hints on how to feed service users who are unable to feed themselves

You may be able to observe this in your work placement.

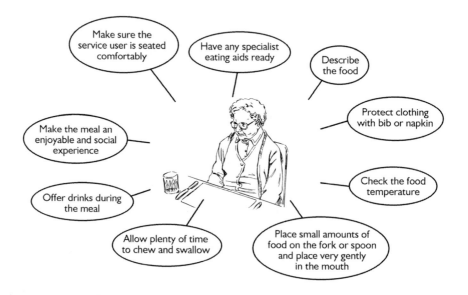

### Safety

- Be aware of the service user's ability to chew and swallow
- Choking is a hazard

- Check the temperature of food and drinks
- Always supervise
- Observe food hygiene rules.

### Take a service user for a short walk.

It is important when planning a walk with a service user that you remember that any help and support must empower the user.

If they do not use a mobility aid, do they need you with them? If they wish to walk about the building or grounds they may be able to do this on their own. You may need to let your supervisor know of the user's wishes in case they fall or become ill while out walking.

If the service user has a mobility aid you must ensure that they are using it in the most appropriate and safe way.

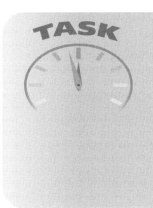

## TASK

### Practical tasks for older service users

Carry out a practical task for an older service user. Carry out a task such as making tea, serving a snack or take a service user for a walk.

When you have carried out the chosen task you must assess your own performance:

1. Look at your strengths – what did you do best?
2. What could you have done better?
3. How did you empower the service user you carried out the task for?

## AO6 Carry out a recreational activity with older service users and assess own performance

Recreation covers a broad range of activities. In this unit you will look at the role of recreation in supporting:

- Physical well-being
- Intellectual well-being
- Social well-being.

### The benefits of recreational activity

Recreational activities are important for health and well-being. You will already be familiar with the ideas of keeping fit to maintain health, but recreation helps to maintain more than just physical health. The role of recreational activities in maintaining intellectual and social well-being is also important. It is useful to consider the three areas of intellectual, social and physical recreational activity.

Recreation can be taken to mean anything that is done as a leisure pursuit. Hobbies are recreational. For some people their paid work may also be an enjoyable recreation. However, for this unit, we will limit recreation to leisure activities. In some cases these may also form part of a therapy. That is, they may be part of a programme to maintain or restore health and well-being – many occupational therapy activities are recreational.

Recreation normally has the emotional benefit that you enjoy doing it. This is a very positive benefit as it fits in with the idea of recreation bringing a balance back to your life. Where work, school or college may be stressful, recreation provides activities that, while being demanding, are also relaxing.

### Physical benefits

Physical activity contributes to fitness in several ways.

- **Strength** – the ability of muscles to work over short periods of time – is required for lifting or the act of jumping
- **Stamina** – the ability for muscles to continue working without fatigue (becoming tired) – is improved
- **Suppleness** – the flexibility of the joints. Exercise to develop suppleness is part of warming up and avoids strains to muscles and joints
- **Speed of reaction** – the ability to respond rapidly to changes. This is linked to things like hand–eye co-ordination. Linked to these are improved balance and agility
- **Heart and lung efficiency** – regular physical recreation makes the heart, lungs and circulation work. Exercise improves these organs' ability to provide oxygen to the body. This has the benefit of reducing the risk of heart disease
- **Determination** – regular physical activity has a knock-on effect by providing the determination to follow tasks through to a finish.

Different physical activities develop different aspects of fitness. Jogging and dancing develop stamina. Gymnastics improves suppleness. Badminton improves strength, suppleness and stamina.

Clearly activities need to be balanced with ability and age. Well-thought-out physical recreation provides benefits to physical health. It is also important to recognise that there are many activities that are not considered to be sports but that also contribute to physical health, such as recreational dancing and walking for pleasure.

### Intellectual benefits

You may think that all your mental activity should be confined to school or college. Recreation should be relaxing. Intellectual activity can, however, provide a stimulating, satisfying and, at the same time, relaxing recreation.

These types of activity often involve problem-solving in some way, for instance in games such as chess.

Reading also provides an intellectual stimulus. Reading for relaxation can involve stories that stimulate your imagination. Using your imagination stimulates mental activity and satisfaction in the enjoyment of the story. Many books also involve problem-solving as part of the enjoyment. Mysteries and detective stories often give sufficient information to enable you to solve the problem before the main characters.

Problem-solving activities and using your imagination both lead to a more active mind. You can use your experiences from reading to help make connections and solve problems for yourself in your life. Strategy games or books that involve thinking about choices help to make you analyse questions, such as 'What would happen if. . .?' This can carry over into your daily activities where you start to think further about the consequences of your actions.

Many hobbies such as collecting, learning new skills (such as playing musical instruments) or making objects (models or pottery) involve intellectual skills. Meeting with others with similar interests in clubs and societies provides some of the social benefits of recreation.

### Social benefits

People are naturally social animals. One of the worst possible tortures is to deprive a person of contact with other people. To be social animals we need to know how to interact with other people.

The need for social contact is recognised in most caring systems. For older people, there is a risk of isolation. Where a husband or wife dies, the surviving partner may be left to live in a house with little contact with other people. This isolation can be worsened by difficulties in moving out of the house. Many social services departments recognise this and organise day centres to support people by coming together for social interaction. Other recreational activities are often provided to support this. Dances, bingo and special swimming sessions for pensioners, for example, can all be provided to help maintain social interaction.

Shared recreational activities imply shared interests. This is the first step towards friendship. The benefits of recreational activities are normally a mixture of physical, intellectual and social. The mixture contributes to a balanced personality and a balanced lifestyle.

## Effects of age

Age has an effect on physical recreation. Some activities require skills and strength to be developed and are most appropriate for people when they are at their fittest, as adolescents and young adults. Such activities may be inappropriate for older people, whose speed of reaction may be reduced.

# 10 Preparing to work with people with disabilities

## To complete this unit you will need to:

- Describe the different types of provision for people with disabilities and explain how the provision meets their needs
- Describe the different types of disability and their effects on service users
- Investigate the accessibility of health or social care or early years services
- Investigate the aids available for people with disabilities
- Plan and carry out a developmental activity with a service user who has a disability
- Evaluate the effectiveness of the activity.

 **AO1**  Describe the different types of provision for people with disabilities and explain how the provision meets their needs

### Introduction

Disability may be either:

- **Physical disability** – such as arthritis, chronic heart disease, muscular dystrophy, multiple sclerosis
- **Sensory disability** – such as blindness, deafness
- **Mental health disabilities**, now more usually referred to as learning difficulty in children – such as Down's syndrome, cerebral palsy or, in older people, Alzheimer's disease.

Some of these disabilities may be inherited, for instance cystic fibrosis or Huntington's chorea.

There are many people who need specific support because of a disability. This includes people with mental and/or physical disabilities.

The purpose of care is to provide the support necessary to enable the individuals to become as independent as possible. For example, many people who are registered blind may spend some time in residential care. There they learn the skills necessary to live safely and with confidence in a society of mostly sighted people.

For some people the disability may be so great that they would find it difficult to cope outside their residential care facility. Their care is planned to enable them to be as independent as possible.

When discussing support services for people with disabilities we need to keep in mind that each person will react differently to the same disability. For this reason we must always regard each service user as an individual and focus on their individual needs, both physical and emotional, rather than on their disability.

For example, some people with disabilities may be able to cope and live at home, while others with the same disability may require much support and may even need residential care.

Any of the services in this section can meet the needs of people with disabilities. In addition to services that are used by everyone, people with disabilities may need specialist services.

*Physiotherapists at work*

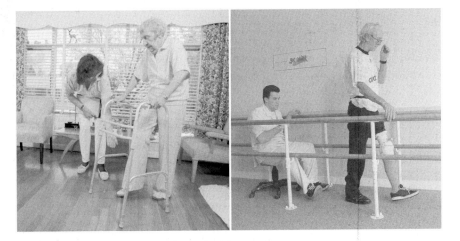

The home situation of people with disabilities varies according to the severity of their disability. Many people with a disability live alone or with their partner; many see no relatives or friends for long periods. Those with severe disabilities are more likely to need domiciliary care from home carers and other support such as meals-on-wheels and visits from an occupational or physiotherapist. They also need regular support from the health visitor and social workers.

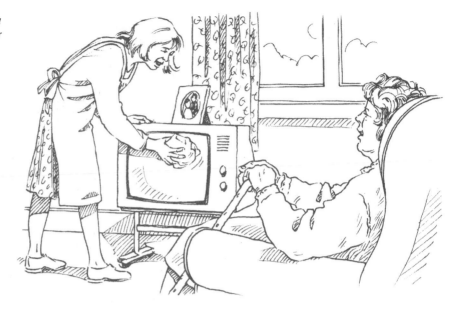

*A home carer with a service user*

Even the simplest illness may assume a great importance for a person with a disability. They may also experience other situations that cause problems such as:

- Mental deterioration
- Loneliness
- Accidents and falls
- Rheumatism/arthritis

- Hearing loss
- Visual defects
- Nutrition problems
- Bronchitis.

## Provision for people with disabilities

The diagram on page 317 shows all the services that could be involved in delivering physical assistance or emotional support to a person with a disability.

As you can see, there are many people involved in providing services and assistance to a person with a disability. All these people must work together to provide the best service possible. It is also important that they co-operate very closely with relatives and friends of the service user.

However, most important of all is that everyone, professional workers and carers, must take into account, and act upon, the wishes of the service user. What the service user wants is the most important thing, not what is available to offer them or what we as carers might think is the best thing for them. It is the person with a disability who must have the final say in what services and support they want.

So that the service user can make informed decisions, the carer should:

- Explain what process they are involved in
- Let the service user put forward their own views
- Agree with the service user what services they would wish

*Services for people with disabilities*

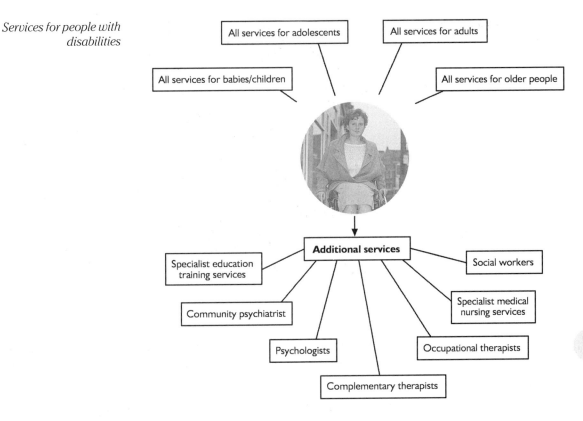

- Talk through with the service user how the services can be delivered
- Involve the service user fully in reviewing the situation as appropriate.

To help you to understand how services for people with disabilities are organised it is important to recognise the four aspects of health and social care:

- Nationally organised health care
- Locally organised health care
- Nationally organised social care
- Locally organised social care.

Clearly, although they work together in many ways, the health services and social services are very different. It is also important to realise that the services can be provided both locally and nationally.

The NHS and the social services form the **statutory sector** of the health and social care services. They are called the statutory services or sector because they were set up by Acts of Parliament (also called statutes) and are funded by public money.

Organisations within the voluntary sector can be very large, like the National Society for the Prevention of Cruelty to Children (NSPCC), or very small local groups that are dealing with a specific need. Voluntary organisations work alongside the statutory services providing care. They can sell their services to a purchaser. This means that the voluntary organisation can be paid by the NHS or the local authority to provide the care.

The case study below shows how the voluntary sector supports service users in the community.

**Case Study**

Sasha had suffered a serious injury and was having to relearn how to move about. Part of her care involved being encouraged to move her legs. To do this required one person to work with her for half an hour at a time.

Sasha's parents were able to do this but they were worried that they would have to give up work and that their other children would suffer. People from the local community heard about the problem and arranged a rota of volunteers to come in each day to work with Sasha.

To make sure that they knew what was necessary, the physiotherapist working with Sasha arranged for all the volunteers to be trained to give the specific support she needed. As a result, Sasha received the therapy necessary. The stress on her family was reduced and, as Sasha improved, her family's life could return to normal.

## Private organisations

Many organisations involved in health and social care charge for their services with the intention of making money. These organisations are part of the **private sector**. The private sector provides services from hospitals and residential homes to individuals working as private nurses, physiotherapists or care assistants in people's own homes.

## Who are the main carers who provide support for people with disabilities?

### General practitioners

The first person that we go to for health care within the community is the general practitioner (GP) or family doctor. GPs are qualified doctors who have undergone further special training. Everyone permanently resident or working in the UK may be registered with a GP. They may select their own GP when they are over 16 years old from the list of GPs kept by the Local Health Authority.

The first port of call for most people requiring health care is the doctor's surgery. The GP:

- Diagnoses (finds out) what is wrong with an individual
- May prescribe treatment, such as medicines.

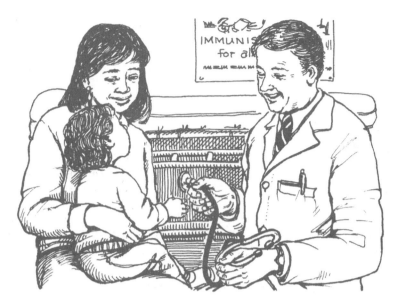

### Health centres

In a health centre you will find:

- **GPs**
- A **practice nurse**
- Services provided by:
    - **Midwives**, who work with pregnant women, may assist the mother during the birth and support mother and child in the days after the birth
    - **Health visitors**, who take over the support of children from midwives – they have a responsibility to do this until the child is 5
    - **Community nurses** (formerly district nurses), who work with people recovering from illness who require health support in their homes – they may be involved in changing dressings on wounds or look after people who are recovering from illness.

Other professionals may also provide services in the health centre, such as:

- **Speech therapist**
- **Occupational therapist**
- **Physiotherapist**
- **Dentist**.

Also based in the community, and developing a more important role following the NHS and Community Care Act, are:

- **Community psychiatric nurses**
- **Community-based mental handicap (RNMH) nurses.**

These nurses provide care for people who have been receiving hospital care, perhaps long-term, and who have now returned to living in the community. They work closely with social workers. Their work is part of the community care that is planned by local authorities.

## People who offer support in hospitals to people with disabilities

Hospitals are traditionally seen as places where people who are too ill to be cared for at home are taken for treatment. They are also the places where people go for operations or for help from a specialist on an outpatient basis.

*Hospital doctor and nurse*

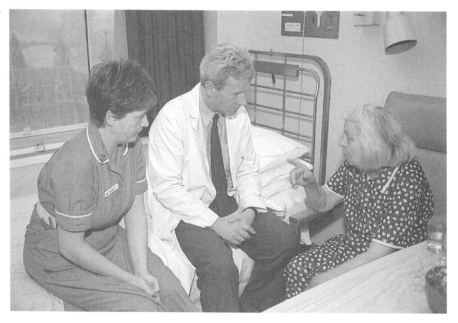

The staff in hospitals include the following.

- **Nurses** carry out the care plan that has been developed by the doctors. Within nursing there are several specialisms, such as nursing sick children, mental health and mental disability.

- **Physiotherapists** help people to improve their ability to move, often helping service users to develop full movement after breaking a bone. They also assist with breathing and treatment routines to help people with cystic fibrosis to clear their lungs.

- **Occupational therapists** (OTs) work to treat illness, both mental and physical, with activity. They work on a one-to-one basis, with groups and with recreational activities. Many OTs work in the community with people with disabilities.

- **Speech therapists** work with people with speech disorders. These range from children with delayed speech development to older people recovering from strokes. Speech therapists work throughout the health service, often going into schools.

## Residential care for people with disabilities

The reasons for people with disabilities entering residential care vary:

- They may be unable to care for themselves
- They may simply wish to live with other people while still maintaining their independence
- They may be recovering from an illness
- It may be to give their families or carers a break.

Because the needs of people with disabilities vary, the types of residential care also vary. Residential care includes:

- **Nursing homes**, which provide care for people needing the support and skills of a nurse. These people may be recovering from illness or in need of regular nursing treatment.
- **Residential homes**, which provide all the necessities for daily living. People in residential homes can be almost self-supporting or may need support for almost all activities.
- **Sheltered accommodation**, which is a form of residential care where individuals take a lot of responsibility for themselves and may be almost totally independent.

## Community-based personal social care for people with disabilities

The aim of a lot of social care is to support a person with a disability living in their own home. The range of workers who provide this support includes the following people:

### Social workers

Home carers offer domiciliary support (home help) for people unable to do things for themselves. This includes home help support for people with disabilities who need someone to do their housework and shopping. But, most important of all, it provides regular company.

Day-care workers work in day-care centres. Many people with disabilities who can be supported at home also benefit from the opportunity of being with others by regularly attending a day-care centre. The day care may be to provide the home-based carer with time to themselves or to go to work.

Supervisory workers in sheltered workshops provide a halfway stage for some people with disabilities. They provide an opportunity for disabled people to learn and develop skills. These may be the skills of daily living or they may be skills associated with employment. Employment in sheltered workshops both provides an income and builds self-confidence in the people working there.

## Support groups and voluntary groups

This covers a range of organisations from major voluntary organisations, such as the Royal National Institute for the Blind, the Disabled Living Foundation or the Disability Alliance, to neighbourhood groups that are formed to support an individual in need of care.

*A volunteer support worker*

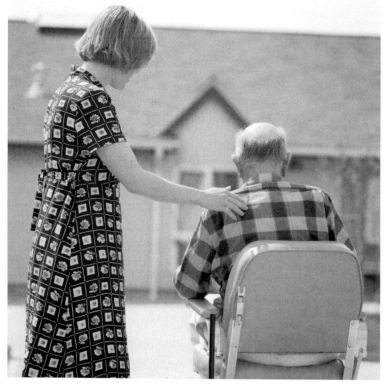

## Early years services for children with disabilities

Early years services for children includes preschool education, such as nurseries and playgroups, which provide important support for young children.

### Day nurseries (private, voluntary and local authority)

Day nurseries look after children under 5. Many are run by Social Services Departments or Education Departments but voluntary groups, private companies or individuals also provide these services.

### Playgroups

Playgroups provide care for children aged between 3 and 5. Some playgroups may take children at the age of 2½ years. Playgroups allow children to learn through playing. A few playgroups are run by local authorities and some look after children with special needs, such as those with physical disabilities.

| Provision | Physical Need | Intellectual Need | Social Need | Emotional Need |
|---|---|---|---|---|
| **Residential homes** | Practical care<br><br>Nursing care<br><br>Food | Games<br><br>Conversation<br><br>Stimulation | Company<br><br>Interaction with staff, residents and visitors | Relationships with staff, carers and visitors<br><br>Empathy from staff<br><br>Support from residents |
| **Resource centre** | Food<br><br>Practical care | Activities | Company<br><br>Interaction with staff, residents and visitors | Relationships with staff, carers and visitors |
| **Special school** | Practical care<br><br>Food | Teaching<br><br>Play<br><br>Activities in class | Interaction with other children, carers and teachers | Relationships with staff, carers and visitors<br><br>Empathy from staff<br><br>Support from other children |
| **Day centre** | Practical care<br><br>Food | Games<br><br>Cards<br><br>Discussions | Interaction with other service users, staff and visitors | Relationships with staff, carers and visitors<br><br>Empathy from staff and service users |
| **Sheltered accommodation** | Housing<br><br>Practical care | Support from warden<br><br>Intellectual activities organised by warden | Interaction with warden, visitors and other carers | Relationships with staff, carers and visitors |

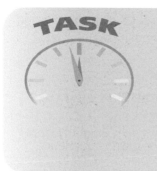

## TASK

### Different types of provision for people with disabilities

Identify in your local community three services that support people with disabilities. The location of these can be identified on a map of the area.

Explain in detail the purpose of this provision and also show how the three services you have selected meet the physical, intellectual, social and emotional needs of the service users.

**Case Study**

Mrs Patel is 76 years old. She is an independent lady but has suffered a stroke at home. Her friend found her, called an ambulance, and she was admitted to hospital.

After a week in hospital the hospital social worker called a meeting of all the people who were looking after her, the doctor, nurses, dietician, physiotherapist and also, most important of all, Mrs Patel was included.

It was hoped that she would go into a residential home (as she could not feed herself or get in and out of her bed or bath) but Mrs Patel felt strongly that she wanted to go back to her own home although the doctor and rest of the team did not agree. However Mrs Patel's wishes had to be taken into account and it was agreed to organise community services to help her live as independent a life as possible in her own home.

It was agreed that she would receive:

- Meals-on-wheels 7 days a week until she could cook her own meals again
- Support from the Community/District nurse
- Support from the occupational therapist to learn how to cook and look after herself again
- Aids to daily living

and that

- A carer would bath her 4 times a week
- A home carer would cook her breakfast and evening meals.

*Describe the methods of referral used in the case study.*

*What aids to daily living would you give to Mrs Patel?*

*What was Mrs Patel's role in the case meeting?*

*Which elements of the care value base have been met in the case study?*

*Describe how the workers in this case empowered Mrs Patel.*

AO2 # Describe the different types of disability and their effects on service users

People of any age may have disabilities but every person with a disability will react differently to it. There are many different types of impairment and people react differently to all of them.

Disabilities can have various consequences for people who experience them.

## Physical disabilities and learning difficulties

### Cerebral palsy

Severely brain-damaged children may suffer from cerebral palsy, which affects the regions of the brain that control movement and muscle tension. It produces stiffness, floppiness, weakness, involuntary movements or unsteadiness. Children with cerebral palsy may have problems with communicating. Electronic communication systems using voice synthesisers and computers have opened up a whole range of opportunities to communicate for people with speech difficulties.

### Hydrocephalus and spina bifida

Spina bifida (split spine) is not on its own a cause of mental disability. Spina bifida is a congenital abnormality caused by the arches of one of the vertebrae not fusing together so that the spine is split in two. The symptoms of spina bifida may include paralysis of the legs, incontinence and mental disability as a result of hydrocephalus (fluid on the brain), which is commonly associated with spina bifida.

### Multiple sclerosis

People with multiple sclerosis experience muscle wastage and will eventually develop mobility problems, which may lead to depression.

### Degenerative diseases

The ageing body is increasingly subject to degenerative diseases. These are diseases that gradually worsen over time and can be any of the following:

- **Atheroma** – a gradual build-up of fatty deposits on the walls of the arteries, giving rise to coronary heart disease and strokes
- **Osteoarthritis** – where changes occur in the joints, giving rise to pain and loss of mobility
- **Brain degeneration** – caused by either Alzheimer's disease, which is the excessive degeneration of the nerve cells, or atheroma of the arteries supplying the brain. Both these conditions can lead to gradual loss of intellectual power and ability

*Access to services*

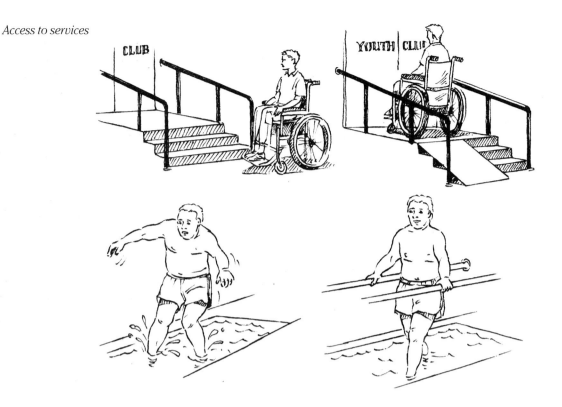

### Effects on service users of not being able to access services and facilities

#### Physical

The inability to access services may affect a person's health – if they cannot get access to services their health may get worse or they might even die.

#### Intellectual

If children do not have access to school their intellectual growth may be affected. They may fail to learn and may leave school without any qualifications.

#### Emotional

Failure to gain access to service may affect a service user's self-esteem. They may feel unwanted and that they are being treated as second-class citizens.

#### Social

Service users may feel isolated if they are unable to overcome barriers to services. Children may have difficult in keeping in touch with friends if they cannot go to the same school.

**Case Study**

Sally is a 10-year-old girl with physical and learning difficulties. She was a very bright and sociable until she had a road accident a year ago, in which she suffered brain damage and also damaged her back. She now has to use a wheelchair.

She had an operation on her brain to remove a blood clot and her back was immobilised so that it could recover from the accident.

While in hospital Sally was looked after by doctors who prescribed medicines, physiotherapists who helped her with movement and social workers who worked with her and her family. An occupational therapist helped Sally's family to decide what adaptations needed to be made to her home to allow her to live there after her discharge from hospital. Sally's social worker also helped her by talking about the accident to her and supporting her in making decisions about her life.

When she was discharged from hospital a community nurse visited to change her dressing and check up on her treatment.

Sally attends her local school where special arrangements have been made to accommodate her disability. Ramps have been built to allow her access to the classrooms and a new toilet has been built for her. She also has the support of a classroom assistant.

Sally is taken to school by a special bus and while in school can call on a special care assistant who helps her go to the toilet.

*What changes have been made in school? Describe these carefully.*

*What aids to daily living do you think Sally will need to live at home?*

*Describe each professional's role and explain the informal care Sally would receive from friends and family.*

## Ways of overcoming barriers

### Adaptations

One important aspect of providing support to any service user is to do so in a way that maintains the service user's independence and dignity.

Aim to:

- Listen and respond to communications from service users

- Information about services available and help people get appropriate support
- Information about assistive equipment
- A visiting service for people, offering companionship
- A good neighbour scheme – visiting, shopping, gardening and other household tasks
- Holidays
- A telephone link – volunteers contact the housebound person with a disability at a pre-arranged time each day to check they are OK and also to offer support
- Day centres
- Coffee shops and luncheon clubs
- Free transport.

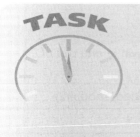

## TASK

### Survey the accessibility of services and facilities for users with disabilities

Choose a health, social care or early years setting and carry out a survey to investigate the accessibility for disabled people to the chosen service.

Describe in detail

1. Barriers to access
2. The effects that these barriers could have on the service user.

Describe how these barriers could be overcome.

 **AO4**  **Investigate the aids available for people with disabilities**

### Why do people with disabilities need help with daily living activities?

The quality of life of a service user will depend to some extent on their being able to move around freely without pain, discomfort or danger. We all take mobility (the ability to walk, wash, dress, feed ourselves, etc.) for granted from the time we first learn to walk.

If a person's mobility is reduced, the scope of their daily lives can become severely limited, as they may be unable to get out of bed, wash or feed themselves. A number of service users need physical assistance with daily living activities, such as eating, walking, hearing or seeing. This support and assistance has to be provided safely and using equipment such as wheelchairs, walking frames and hearing aids where necessary.

## The types of aid available to help people with disabilities

How can the use of assistive equipment help a dependent person to live as independent a life as possible in their own home? Assistive equipment improves the service user's ability to carry out certain tasks such as feeding and bathing. It can also make life easier for staff and service users in residential establishments.

The range of equipment available to the dependent person, either in their own home or in residential care, is vast. It ranges from knives and forks to large and very expensive pieces of equipment, such as hoists and stairlifts. However simple the aid, the purpose is to help the disabled person to move about or carry out daily living tasks as well as they can.

### The categories of assistive equipment

Assistive equipment falls into the following categories:

- Personal care support
- Hoists and lifting equipment
- Eating and drinking aids
- Help with dressing and undressing
- Mobility aids
- Reading and hearing aids.

### Personal care support for people with disabilities

This includes such aids as rails in bathrooms, showers and toilets, also commodes, bedpans, urinals and waste disposal units.

Using a rubber mat in the bath can prevent the service user from slipping. Hand rails allow the service user to walk unaided in bathrooms or toilets. The rail also allows the person with a disability to lower themselves on to the toilet. Sometimes a raised toilet seat also helps.

A bath seat allows the person to swing themselves, on their own, into a bath or shower, thus not stripping them of their dignity or self-respect.

### Hoists and lifting equipment

Hoists and lifting equipment not only help maintain the independence of the service user but are also an enormous help to the carers. They make lifting safer and easier. Some hoists are fixed, perhaps beside a person's bed or bath, but most are portable. This means that they can be used in a number of situations in the home with safety. They may be either manually or electrically operated.

### Eating and drinking aids

To help people feed themselves, there are a number of aids available: cutlery, plates, trays, drinking aids. For example, service users with arthritis of the hand, which may cause poor grip, can have knives and forks with thick handles. Plates with rubber bases to stop the plate from slipping are useful for people with the use of only one hand.

### Help with dressing and undressing

People with disabilities sometimes have problems with dressing and undressing. These are simple tasks but can be made difficult by even the simplest disability, such as a broken finger or a muscle strain. Arthritic joints make it difficult to do up buttons or lift arms above the head. Service users can use Velcro instead of zips or buttons. A number of aids to dressing can be used, as illustrated in the figure on page 82.

### Mobility aids

Getting around the house or residential home can cause problems for many disabled or elderly people. Help can be available in the form of a simple walking stick or walking frame.

Wheelchairs can be either electrically or manually propelled.

Buildings can be adapted to help people. For example, kitchen worktops can be lowered to allow wheelchair users to access them. Ramps can be installed so that people can get in and out of buildings.

For people who need extra support when walking, a variety of sticks are available (see page 89). They are usually made from aluminium and can be adjusted in length or folded. Variations include tripod and quadruped sticks, which provide extra stability, and traditional wooden sticks are still popular. Seat sticks are useful. These are made of lightweight aluminium and can be turned into a seat when the user wants to rest for short periods.

For people who are unable to bear their own weight or who need extra support when walking, a range of lightweight, aluminium elbow crutches are available. Their height can be adjusted to suit the individual. It is important that service users and carers should understand the correct way to use crutches and a physiotherapist will usually advise on this.

### Reading and hearing aids

For people with arthritis of the fingers or wrist, help is available in the form of page turners and writing aids. Those with sight problems can obtain reading glasses or computer programmes that create large type that partially sighted people can read. Talking books and large print books are also available.

### Bed comfort

Although service users are encouraged to get up and to be as mobile as possible there will always be situations where they spend considerable periods of time in bed or sitting in a chair. Comfort can be improved by using:

- Pillows to give extra support (triangular pillows are often used)
- Backrests to give support when sitting upright in bed
- Bed cradles to protect or take the weight of bedclothes
- Rings and cushions to sit on
- Fleecy pads to protect buttocks, elbows and heels
- Ladder hoists, which consist of a simple arrangement allowing service users to pull themselves into a sitting position when in bed or in the bath
- Trapeze lifts to help service users to move in bed or in the bath.

Remember that as a learner you would not use any of these items without help and advice from your supervisor.

### Bathroom aids

A vast array of equipment is available to assist service users and carers with washing and bathing. Examples include:

- Special showers and baths
- Safety rails
- Bath seats
- Mobile shower chairs
- Grip bath and shower mats
- Safety rails
- Bath seat
- Toilet aids
- Grip mat.

When service users are confined to bed, bedpans and urinals may have to be used. This is not ideal and whenever possible the service user should be taken to the lavatory or use a commode. Equipment available includes:

- Special toilet seats
- Raised seats
- Inflatable toilet seats
- Sahichairs.

### Aids to help with eating and drinking

Many disabled and elderly people you will meet during your work experience are helped to maintain independence when eating and drinking using a variety of devices including:

- Special cutlery
- Feeding cups
- Plate guards
- Automatic feeders.

## Sources for obtaining aids

### Statutory

A range of aids are available from the local social services or health authority. Aids such a walking sticks, crutches, and wheelchairs are available on loan for as long as the service user needs them.

### Private

A number of private organisations specialise in the provision of aids and adaptations, which can be purchased. Look in the Yellow Pages for a list of these organisations in your area.

### Voluntary organisations/associations

Voluntary organisation play a large part in the provision of aids and adaptations and a number of them specialise in certain areas – for example providing special aids for the hearing-impaired or the blind.

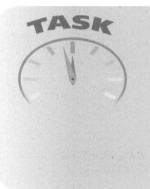

## TASK

### Use of a range of aids for people with disabilities

Investigate three aids that are available for people with disabilities. These should include one aid used to help with mobility, one to help with sensory impairment and one to improve daily living.

Describe how these aids are used, their purpose and where service users can get them.

Write a guide for service users on how to use these aids.

 **AO5** 

## Plan and carry out a developmental activity with a service user who has a disability

### How to choose a developmental activity

To help you decide what developmental activity you might carry out you should have a long discussion with an individual service user. Remember that the service user's wishes and needs come first and that any thing you do must not disempower them. Discuss your ideas with the service user and select one activity that you are both happy with.

Having a long discussion helps to overcome the problems of making decisions too quickly or doing things in a certain way just because that is the way it is always done.

## Plan the activity

Planning is an important part of carrying out any task or activity. When you have selected an activity, you will need to consider how long you have been given to carry it out and whether you can fit in with all the other work you have to do on this course. **Never begin a developmental activity with a service user unless you can complete it.**

To help you decide what activity to chose you should have a long discussion with your teacher. Remember that the service user's wishes and needs come first and that any thing you do must not disempower them or their carers.

### Drawing up a plan for the appropriate activity

Planning is an important part of carrying out any task, activity or plan. When you have identified the appropriate activity, you will need to consider how long you have been given to carry out the plan. Remember the activity must be one that is creative, able to develop a skill or is therapeutic.

The plan must include:

- The aims of the activity (creative, develop a skill or therapeutic)
- Objectives of the plan
- Resources needed
- Timescales
- Cost
- Targets of the activity.

The health and safety issues relating to the activity must also be considered.

You must set the preset criteria for measuring the success of the activity (for example, if it is to develop a skill such as using a hoist safely, what criteria would you set? Would the preset criteria be different if it was a creative activity you had set?)

The care values must also be considered

- How will you promote equality and diversity?
- How will you maintain confidentiality?
- How will you make sure that you promote the individual's rights?
- How will you take into account the individual's beliefs?

## AO6  Evaluate the effectiveness of the activity

### Review of your activity

1. **What have you done so far?**

   - Have you a written record of your activities?

   - Have you and the service user agreed on the activity to be undertaken?

   - Is the activity plan going as you would have hoped?

2. **What needs to be done to put the activity into action?**

   - How can you overcome any problems that you have identified in part 1 above?

   - Do you and the service user want to make any changes to the plan?

   - What resources will you both need to continue?

### Health and safety considerations involved in the activity

When working in the health and social care services, we must always make sure that what we do does not make it hazardous for either the service user or ourselves. You must, therefore, take into consideration any health and safety factors of the activity you are organising. Read Unit 4 again before you start the activity. It will give you a basic understanding of health and safety procedures.

When planning the developmental activity, remember to examine and identify any common hazards that could occur.

Is the environment safe? Make sure that any equipment or accommodation you use is safe. In particular, consider:

- First aid equipment

- Safety precautions (fire or evacuation procedures, etc.)

- Safe working practices (fire guards, etc.)

- Alarms and emergency systems, such as fire alarms.

- Whether any equipment (e.g. wheelchair or hoist) is safe and in good working order.

### How to review the activity

When you have completed the activity, you will need to review your own individual performance against the tasks that you agreed to undertake with the service user. To review the activity you will first need to look at whether you carried out the agreed activity. You should look at:

- Whether the service user has benefited from the activity

- Whether or not resources were used effectively

- Whether you dealt with any problems effectively
- Whether you maintained the health and safety of those you were working with.

### Review of your performance

To do this, you will need to look back at your original activity plan.

When reviewing what you have done, it often a very good idea to ask the person you did the activity with – the service user – what they thought about it.

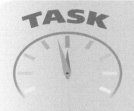

**TASK**

## Carry out a developmental activity with a service user who has a disability and asses your own performance

Carry out an appropriate developmental activity for a service user. This activity can be a game of cards, writing a letter or painting.

You must individually:

1. Plan – the aim of the activity – objectives – resources – time scale – cost
2. Set the criteria for measuring the success of the activity
3. Carry out
4. Monitor and
5. Review

the selected activity.

You will need to consider the:
a. Medical needs and
b. Care needs

of the service user and also

c. Health and safety issues.

It is also very important that you consider how you can involve the service user in planning the activity so as to empower them.

When you have carried out the chosen task you must assess your own performance:

1. Look at your strengths – what did you do best
2. What could you have done better?
3. How did you empower the service user?

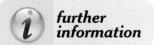

**further information**

Bell L (1999) *Care Fully. A Handbook for Home Care Assistants.* Age Concern, London

Clarke L (2000) *Health and Social Care for Intermediate GNVQ.* Nelson Thornes, Cheltenham

Clarke L (2002) *Health and Social Care GCSE*. Nelson Thornes, Cheltenham

Nolan Y (1998) *Care. NVQ Level 2 Student Handbook*. Heinemann, Oxford

Nolan Y (2003) *S/NVQ Level 3 Promoting Independence*. Heinemann, Oxford

Worsley I (1999) *Taking Good Care. A Handbook for Home Care Assistants*. Age Concern, London

www.bda-dyslexia.org.uk – British Dyslexia Association

www.disabilityalliance.org.uk – Disability Alliance

www.dlf.org.uk – The Disabled Living Foundation

www.rnib.org.uk – Royal National Institute for the Blind

www.rnid.org.uk – Royal National Institute for the Deaf

www.scope.org.uk – SCOPE

## Summary

- There are different types of provision for people with different types of disability, for example community psychiatric nurses, physiotherapists in a hospital setting and day-care workers in day-care centres.

- There are many different types of disability and each will affect a service user differently.

- Access to services ranges from self-referral to compulsory referral but carers should be aware that barriers to gaining access can exist if information is poor regarding what services are available.

- To help people with disabilities a range of aids is available, such as walking frames, hearing aids, hand rails for staircases and special cutlery.

- When carrying out a developmental activity with a service user who has a disability, it should be carefully planned, recorded and reviewed. The service user should also be asked for their feedback.

# Practical first aid in care settings

## To complete this unit you will need to:

- Conduct out a risk assessment and review health and safety for a care setting
- Assess the scene of an accident and make the area safe
- Assess a casualty for signs of consciousness
- Understand and perform ABC procedure
- Demonstrate and understand the correct first aid procedure for dealing with an unconscious casualty who is breathing and has a pulse and for an unconscious casualty who is not breathing and has no pulse
- Use correct procedures to call for help
- Demonstrate and understand the correct first aid procedures when dealing with asthma and choking
- Demonstrate and understand the correct first aid procedures when dealing with bleeding, including wounds where there is an embedded object
- Demonstrate and understand the correct first aid procedure when dealing with burns
- Demonstrate and understand the correct first aid procedure when dealing with a casualty in shock

**AO1** **Conduct out a risk assessment and review health and safety for a care setting**

### Potential hazards in care settings

Going to work for the first time, or going to your first real work experience, can be exciting and a bit strange. It can also be dangerous. Every year over 500 people in the UK die at work and several hundred thousand have to stay off work because of injury.

Some hazards cannot be seen, such as:

- Stress
- Radiation
- Inadequate information as to the moving and handling of service users.

Some health hazards may affect workers slowly over many years, such as the effects of working down coal-mines or working with asbestos.

## What can you do about hazards in care settings?

Organisations (such as factories, colleges , hospitals and the one you work in) will usually have:

- A health and safety officer, who will have the overall responsibility for putting the organisation's health and safety policy into practice
- A system for reporting defects in equipment
- An accident book for recording details about accidents and injuries.

A basic function of all care organisations is to provide a safe and controlled environment for staff, service users and visitors. The wide-ranging nature of care organisations means that each organisation has its own particular requirements in terms of health and safety. For example, nurseries or playgroups have different requirements from a home for elderly people. Each will also have its own particular hazards.

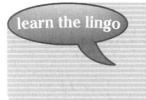

A **hazard** is something that can cause harm, including ill-health and injury.

The **risk** is the chance, however high or low, that you, a service user or a visitor may be harmed by the hazard.

The hazard presented by a substance (chemicals, bleach) is its potential to cause harm. It may make you cough, damage your liver or even kill you. Some substances can harm you in several different ways, e.g. if you breathe them in, swallow them or get them on your skin.

The risk from a substance or article is the likelihood that it will harm you when you do not use it properly in the workplace. Poor control can create a risk, even from a substance that is not very hazardous (e.g. bleach or soap). However, with proper precautions, the risk of being harmed by even the most hazardous substance can be adequately controlled.

Below is a list of hazards to look out for:

- Unguarded or unsupervised equipment
- Slippery or broken walkways
- Loose or broken wiring

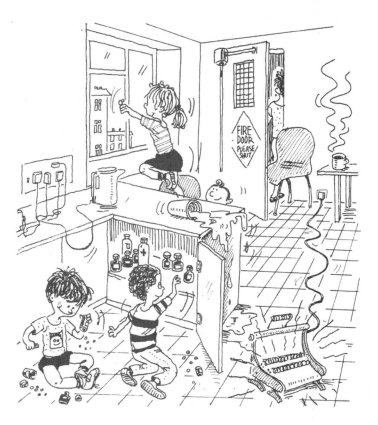

- Poor lighting
- Leaks of water or gas
- Blocked doors and emergency fire exits
- Poor signing (fire exit, etc.)
- Unhygienic toilets and slippery surfaces
- Broken tiles and mirrors
- Inadequate storage for cleaning materials
- Poorly maintained lifts and elevators.

### Safety features to reduce hazards (Safety Audit)

Hygiene and welfare

This includes:

- Separate marked toilets for each sex
- Toilets kept clean and in working order and ventilated
- Wash basin with hot and cold running water
- Soap, dryers and nail-brushes where appropriate
- Waste bins regularly emptied
- Facilities for taking food and drink

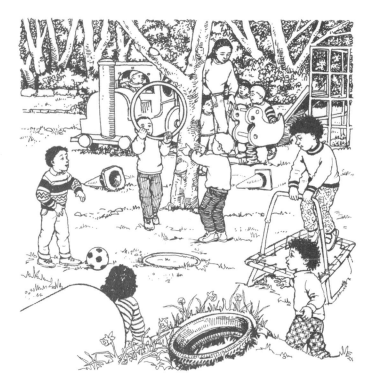

- Safe methods for handling, storing and transporting materials
- Drugs stored and used in such a way as to minimise risk to health.

## Comfort

The employer should consider the comfort and safety of employees, including:

- Making sure furniture is placed so that sharp corners do not present a danger to staff or service users
- Providing good ventilation in bathrooms, toilets, bedrooms
- Providing a thermometer in each work room so that staff can check temperature – this is important in areas where elderly people are cared for, and also for babies and young children
- Installing good lighting.

## Cleanliness

The employer should ensure that:

- Workplace, furniture and fittings are kept clean
- All rubbish and waste food are regularly removed
- All spillages are cleaned up immediately
- Dirty linen is stored appropriately
- Dressings and medicines are disposed of according to instructions.

If a new cleaning product is introduced, an employer is obliged to tell employees of any possible harmful effects.

# Safety Audit

## Safe procedures of work

Systems of work can affect your health and the service user's health. For example, do you know what would happen to your work clothes if you were splashed by a chemical you were using to clean a floor?

Could poor design of working areas like bathrooms lead to backache?

Are you aware of any potential safety hazard? Is there any risk of service users or patients transmitting disease? If you were working with old, unchecked electrical appliances in a service user's home, would you know of the dangers or to whom to report your concerns? Are all students and staff aware of the procedures for staff who are vulnerable to physical violence?

## Example of Safety Audit (survey): How could you help prevent fire?

The answers to all the following questions should be 'yes'.

- Are all parts of the premises clear of waste and rubbish, particularly:
  - Storerooms?
  - Attics and basements?
  - Boiler rooms and other equipment rooms?
  - The bottoms of lift shafts?
  - Staircases and under the stairs?
- Smoking:
  - Are enough ashtrays provided in all the areas where smoking is permitted?
  - Have staff been warned to use the ashtrays and not to throw cigarettes or matches into wastepaper bins, through gratings or out of windows?
- Electricity:
  - Do all parts of the electrical installation comply with the Institute of Electrical Engineers (IEE) regulations for electrical installations?
  - Is the electrical installation inspected and tested at least every five years?
  - Are staff trained to report frayed leads and faulty equipment?
- If you do not have central heating:
  - Are heating appliances fixed rather than portable?
  - Are they provided with adequate and secure fireguards?

11

● Have the staff been warned to keep combustible materials away from heaters?

## Legislation and regulations

The Heath and Safety at Work Act 1974 is the law that controls health and safety in the workplace. Both employers and employees (you) have responsibilities under this law to protect the health and safety of yourselves and other people.

### *Some of the more important responsibilities of the employer*

An employer must provide a workplace that is safe from hazards and does not harm an employee's health. This includes:

● Having a safety policy
● Hygiene and welfare
● Comfort
● Cleanliness.

Safety policy

Employers must tell their staff how they are going to ensure their health and safety. This is called a safety policy. It should tell you:

● Who your key managers are, so that you can report any unsafe situation
● How they intend to protect you at work, including rules for safe procedures when carrying out particular tasks.

The safe procedure rules will cover, for example:

● The control of infection
● The wearing of protective clothing
● Using correct moving and handling procedures
● Training in the use of equipment.

The safety policy will, in many cases, be in the form of a booklet, or it may perhaps be a notice on a notice board. The document should also be published in a number of languages to make it accessible to all staff.

A manager of a residential home for elderly people, for example, or of a day centre for children must ensure that all staff know their duties so that they pay appropriate attention to health and safety when they carry out their work.

The maintenance of a safe environment and the practice of safe procedures enables the service user to feel secure and confident. That is one of the necessities of good social care. Make sure you know the safety rules and obey them.

## The Manual Handling Operations Regulations 92

These regulations came into effect on 1 January 1993. They place the responsibility for the safety of workers on the management of the organisation you are working for. All employers must ensure the safety of their workers in the following ways:

- All manual handling tasks that might injure anyone should be avoided where possible. If it is not possible to avoid a hazardous manual handling task, it must be assessed first to decide how it is to be done.
- Once the task has been assessed, action must be taken to reduce the risk of injury.

The employer must ensure that they have a safe manual handling policy and must give training before staff begin lifting.

As a care worker, you too should always be aware of the appropriate and safe way to carry out a manual handling task. You should also call for assistance when you think it is necessary.

There are some special difficulties with lifting service users:

- Many service users are too heavy to be moved bodily
- Service users are unwieldy and difficult to grasp
- Many dependent or injured service users make unexpected movements
- Most injuries occur to care staff because of the physical behaviour of the service user.

Things to look for when assessing a proposed moving task:

- Does the service user need to be moved?
- Could the service user move themselves?
- Could a lifting aid be used?
- How long will it take to move the service user?

## First aid boxes

Employees should have access to a first aid box whilst at work. First aid boxes should be easily identifiable and accessible throughout the workplace. The box should not be locked and anyone who is injured should be treated by an appointed person, i.e. someone who is appointed to take charge when there is an injury.

The first aider responsible for the box should be notified to ensure that the stock is replenished.

There is no mandatory list of items that should be included in a first aid box. The required minimum level of first-aid equipment is a suitably stocked and properly identified first-aid container. Such a container should be provided in an easily accessible location.

information is available on their websites (www.redcross.org.uk and www.sja.org.uk).

## Priorities in an emergency

The key thing in an emergency situation is to help the victims as quickly as possible without making the situation worse or putting anyone else (including yourself!) at risk.

You should:

- Stay calm
- Assess the situation for risks to yourself and the victim
- Ensure safety for yourself, the casualty and other helpers
- Establish the condition of the victim (if possible)
- Get help
- Only move the casualty if there is a risk of further injury to them.

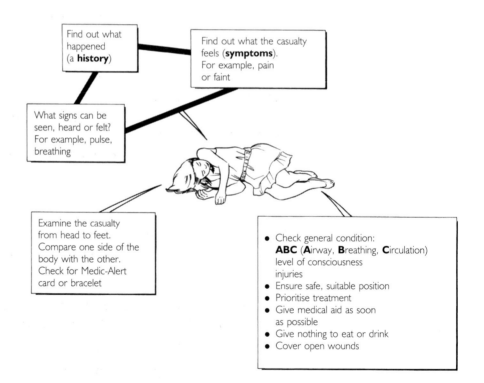

Find out what happened (a **history**)

Find out what the casualty feels (**symptoms**). For example, pain or faint

What signs can be seen, heard or felt? For example, pulse, breathing

Examine the casualty from head to feet. Compare one side of the body with the other. Check for Medic-Alert card or bracelet

- Check general condition: **ABC** (**A**irway, **B**reathing, **C**irculation) level of consciousness injuries
- Ensure safe, suitable position
- Prioritise treatment
- Give medical aid as soon as possible
- Give nothing to eat or drink
- Cover open wounds

## Dangers to the casualty and first aider

There are many possible emergency situations in which a casualty may need first aid. The situation or the accident may vary but the aims for the first aider are always the same. The first aider will not be much help if they become a casualty themselves.

Aims:

- To preserve life (casualty and first aider)
- To prevent the deterioration of the casualty
- To promote recovery.

The first aider may not be able to do any of these if he/she is unable to take action that does not place themself or the casualty in danger.

## Safety of the first aider

To keep himself or herself from any danger the first aider must keep calm and try to understand what has happened. First aiders must not approach the scene if it is not safe to do so (for example, if there is a fire or loose and live electrical wires about the scene).

The first aider must make a decision as to whether:

- There is any continuing danger (electricity, gas, chemicals, etc)
- The casualty's life is in immediate danger
- There is anyone else about who could help.

## Make the area safe

It is important that you, as a first aider, remain safe and that you try to reduce the risk to yourself and the casualty posed by any hazards in the immediate area. If there is a continuing danger from hazards (such as spilt chemicals, gas, etc) you need to reduce the risk they pose and make the area as safe as possible, for example, switch off the electricity or gas at the mains. Protective clothing may have to be worn before you approach a casualty who has suffered a chemical accident so that you do not contaminate yourself.

The rule for making an area safe is always to try and remove the danger or hazard from the casualty, where possible, and only try to remove the casualty as a last resort.

### Example: Making the area and casualty safe – if you find someone who has suffered an electric shock

- Switch off the current at the mains
- Switch off at the plug or try to pull the plug out
- Do not directly touch the casualty – you will also get a shock
- If you cannot switch off the electric current, break the electric contact by pulling the casualty away from it. Do this by putting a rope around their arm or legs. You must do this without physically touching the casualty yourself
- When pushing the casualty away, stand or kneel on a dry rug, rubber mat or pile of newspapers

● It may be easier to push the contact (wire or equipment) away from the casualty. Do this with a broom handle after insulating your hands with rubber gloves or a dry cloth.

### AO3  Assess a casualty for signs of consciousness

Check airway, breathing and circulation (A, B, C).

Check for unconsciousness.

Check for severe bleeding.

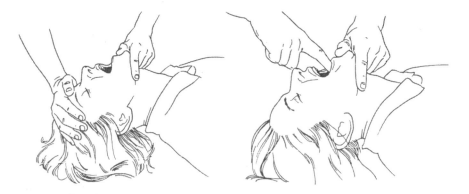

1. Check that the **airway** is clear and keep it open.

2. Check that the casualty is **breathing**. Watch the rise and fall of the chest. Listen for breath.

3. Check for **circulation**, i.e. that the heart is beating. Check for the pulse (heart beat) at the wrist (the radial pulse) and in the neck (the carotid pulse). Use two fingers (not your thumb) and feel for 10 seconds to decide whether the pulse is present or not.

4. Check whether the casualty is **conscious**. See if you can make the person respond to you. Touch them, speak to them, call their name. A casualty who is unconscious will not respond to you. A casualty may

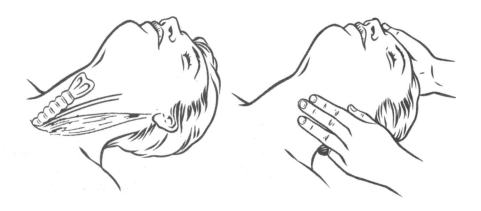

be partially conscious, possibly moving slightly or moaning. You can assess the level of responsiveness using the following code:

A = Alert

V = Responds to voice

P = Responds to pain

U = Unconscious (no response)

5. Place the casualty in the **recovery position** (but if you suspect a spinal or neck injury, do not move the casualty). To do this you turn the casualty on to their side to prevent them choking on saliva or vomit and to prevent the tongue from falling back and blocking the air passages. You should:

a. Kneel beside the casualty

b. Open the airway

c. Remove glasses and fragile objects from the casualty's pockets

d. Place the arm of the casualty nearest to you at right angles to the casualty's body with the elbow bent and the palm uppermost

e. Bring the arm furthest away from you across the chest so that the palm rests against the casualty's cheek

f. Grasp the casualty's far thigh and pull the knee up, keeping the foot flat against the ground

g. With the casualty's hand still pressed to their cheek, pull the far thigh towards you to roll them towards you on to their side

h. Tilt the head back to keep the airway open (you may have to adjust the position of the hand under the cheek)

i. Ensure that the hip and knee of the upper leg are bent at right angles

j. Monitor the breathing and pulse every 10 minutes (write down your observations if possible)

k. Do not give food or fluids.

## What if the casualty isn't breathing?

Do you know? – a person can live for:

- Four weeks without food
- Four days without water
- Only four minutes without oxygen.

If someone stops breathing, you must act quickly. A person who suffers **respiratory arrest** (stops breathing) will very quickly lose consciousness. When breathing stops the patient will suffer **cardiac**

11

**arrest** (the heart will stop beating) within 3–4 minutes. If resuscitation is not started immediately, brain death will occur. We will see later that the main way of resuscitating someone who has stopped breathing is with cardiopulmonary resuscitation (CPR).

**AO4** ## Understand and perform ABC procedure

### What is the ABC rule?

This is a very important rule for first aiders to remember. Thinking of the letters A B C – **A**irway, **B**reathing, **C**irculation – will help you to remember the right order in which to do things in an emergency.

If the airway, breathing and pulse are OK, you can then check for other injuries, such as fractures, cuts, wounds, etc.

### How do you make sure the airway is open?

With the person lying on their back tilt their forehead backwards by placing one hand underneath the neck and the other hand on the forehead. This will ensure that the chin moves upwards.

Remove your hand from under the person's neck and lift the chin upwards and forwards. The mouth will open slightly and the nostrils of the nose will be pointing upwards. In this position the tongue will move from the back of the throat and unblock the air passage.

Once you have unblocked the airway and the person is breathing, you must place them in either of these positions:

- **The prone position** – 'prone' means face downwards and the elbows bent, so that the forearms and hands are under the forehead.
- **The recovery position** – the casualty is lying on their side, with their cheek touching the ground and their face turned slightly towards the ground. This position keeps the airway open and allows any fluid to drain from the mouth.

If the casualty has to be kept in the recovery position for more than 30 minutes, they should be turned on to the opposite side – injuries permitting.

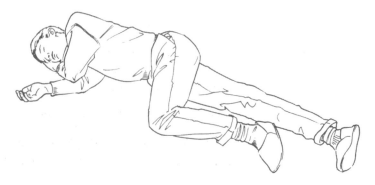

**AO5** **Demonstrate and understand the correct first aid procedure for dealing with an unconscious casualty who is breathing and has a pulse and for an unconscious casualty who is not breathing and has no pulse**

### Correct first aid for dealing with an unconscious casualty who is not breathing

If the person is semi-conscious or unconscious you should also try and measure their level of consciousness.

#### Monitoring levels of consciousness

Unconsciousness can be caused by anything that interrupts the normal working of the brain. The most common causes are:

- Suffocation
- Shock
- Heart attack
- Head injuries
- Poisoning
- Epilepsy and diabetic emergencies.

Levels of consciousness are categorised as follows:

- **Fully conscious** – alert, responds to conversation in normal manner
- **Drowsy** – responds easily but may give muddled or slow answers to questions
- **Semi-conscious** – aroused with difficulty, may only be able to carry out simple activities like moving an arm or leg or fingers, will be aware of pain
- **Unconscious** – no response, no reaction to questions or to pain.

#### Keeping the airway open

Because a person's muscles are usually completely relaxed when they are unconscious they are at particular risk of choking. This is caused by the tongue falling backwards and blocking the air passage. This is one of the first things to look for in an unconscious person. So that air and oxygen can get to the brain, the first thing to do is to make sure that the airway is open.

#### Mouth-to-mouth resuscitation

The brain needs oxygen in order to function. The respiratory (breathing) system relies on our ribs, diaphragm, heart and lungs working together to transport oxygen from the air we breathe to the brain.

A person who is not breathing, therefore, is being starved of oxygen.

If the brain is starved of oxygen for more than 4 minutes it may be permanently damaged. One way to get air to someone's lungs is by breathing into their lungs. This is called **artificial respiration** or **mouth-to-mouth resuscitation**.

The air you breathe into the casualty's lungs will not be as rich in oxygen as the air they would normally breathe but it will be enough to maintain life and avoid brain damage.

### How to do mouth-to-mouth resuscitation

Artificial respiration will do the unconscious person no harm, so don't waste time sending for help. The casualty will die if the brain does not get oxygen immediately.

1. Lie the casualty flat on their back. Open the airway.

2. Close the casualty's nose by pinching it, otherwise the air will escape through the nose.

3. Take a deep breath and put your mouth over the casualty's mouth.

4. Blow into the lungs and watch to observe if the lungs rise. The chest should rise as the air enters the lungs.

5. Carry on blowing into the lungs until the casualty starts to breathe again, or until professional help arrives. Don't blow too hard – just enough to make the chest rise.

6. As soon as the casualty starts to breathe again, put them in the recovery position.

7. With small children or babies, put your mouth over both their nose and their mouth and blow gently into the lungs until the chest rises.

## Ways of treating the casualty with dignity and respect

It is important that you preserve the dignity of the casualty at all times. You should act to provide privacy for the casualty by requesting any onlookers to move back. Providing temporary screens with clothing or a rug or blankets will offer privacy.

The casualty may be unconscious but it is important that you maintain their privacy and dignity at all times.

## Correct first aid for dealing with an unconscious casualty who is not breathing and has no pulse

### Cardiopulmonary resuscitation (CPR)

First, the airway is cleared, then the rescuer blows air into the casualty's lungs. External heart compressions are applied to keep the blood circulating and carrying oxygen to vital organs.

Look carefully at the figure on page 361, which shows how to assess a casualty's breathing. Do not attempt to administer CPR unless you have been taught how to do it properly. This is vital, as it is not a technique that

*How to access a casualty's breathing*

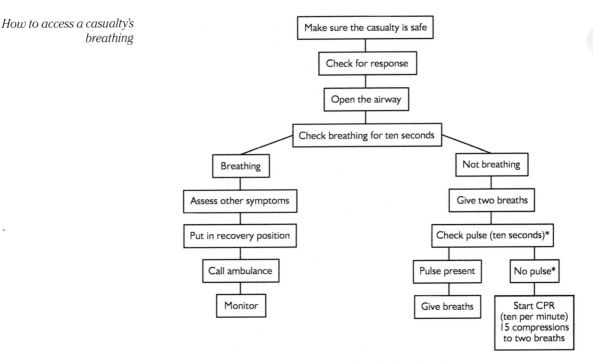

* Compressions may be commenced without checking the pulse.

can be learned from reading a book. Nor is it enough to have seen it done on TV! You need skilled instruction and opportunities to practise using special models.

Send a helper to call an ambulance at once, or, if you are alone, resuscitate for one minute before calling an ambulance.

**All these techniques need to be demonstrated by skilled first aiders and practised regularly.**

When a casualty has no pulse, it means that the heart has stopped beating. To restore the circulation, it is necessary to give chest massage (also known as chest compressions or heart massage).

Chest massage is best done combined with mouth-to-mouth resuscitation. This is called cardiopulmonary resuscitation or CPR. It can be done either by one or two first aiders – one to give mouth-to-mouth ventilation and the other to do chest massage – but note that this procedure can be quite tiring.

How to do chest massage:

1. Lie the casualty flat on their back. Open the airway (see above).

2. Find the correct position for your hands.

3. Leaning over the casualty, with your arms straight, press down vertically on the breastbone to depress it about 4–5cm. Release the pressure without removing your hands. Compression and release should take an equal amount of time.

11

4. Continue giving compressions at a rate of about 100 per minute. Check the pulse after every 10 compressions.

For babies, place the tips of two fingers in a position just below the midpoint of an imaginary line between the nipples. Give chest compressions of about 1.5–2.5cm at a rate of 100 per minute.

With children under 5, put one hand in the same position as you would for an adult. Give compressions of about 2.5–3.5cm at a rate of 100 per minute. For children over 5, use the same method as for adults.

### AO6 Use correct procedures to call for help

In most cases, getting help will involve calling the emergency services. Keep calm and speak slowly and clearly, bearing the following points in mind:

- If possible, use a land line. If you are cut off, the operator will then be able to trace your whereabouts.
- Dial 999 or 112 (on a mobile phone) and state the service required – ambulance, fire or police.
- Give your telephone number.
- State clearly where the casualty is.
- Say exactly what has happened, the number of casualties and the nature of their injuries.

### AO7 Demonstrate and understand the correct first aid procedures when dealing with asthma and choking

#### Asthma

##### What is asthma?

We usually do not think of how we breathe, as it is a passive and effortless procedure. To understand asthma, we must first understand how we breathe.

When someone has forced, wheezy and difficult breathing it is called asthma. The breathing tubes (bronchioles) become narrowed so that it is difficult to breathe out naturally. Some people feel a great weight across their chest and have difficulty in breathing and they may make wheezing noises. During an attack the air passages go into spasm and there is excretion of thick, sticky mucus in the lungs which further reduces the air passages. Breathing in is often normal but only partial breathing out can be achieved during an attack.

### What causes asthma?

Asthma is often an allergic condition. People may be allergic to:

- Pollens
- Smoke
- Animals
- Certain foods.

Sometimes, if a person is worried their asthma can be made worse. Attacks usually occur suddenly and more commonly at night or the early hours of the morning.

### How can you help someone who has an attack of asthma?

If the person is lying down, sit them up (in bed or in a chair) in a comfortable position. In many cases, the person themselves will know which position is most comfortable. Sometimes the person suffering cannot bear to be touched and may want all their clothes loosened. Lean them slightly forward. In this position it is easier to use the chest muscles for breathing. Make sure that there is plenty of fresh air available.

If this is a first attack, a doctor or ambulance should be called.

If the person knows that they suffer from asthma, find out whether they have their inhaler with them. If so, help them to use it. If the medication has no effect within 5 minutes take the sufferer to hospital or dial 999.

Give plenty of reassurance until a doctor or ambulance arrives.

The person will often be very frightened because they are having difficulty in breathing and feel they are suffocating. Young children may panic and will need lots of reassurance and emotional support.

## Choking

Any foreign body (perhaps a fishbone or piece of food) that lodges or sticks in the throat or in the windpipe will cause choking. With children or elderly people the most common cause is food or drink 'going down the wrong way'. With small children, choking is a particular hazard, because of their habit of putting everything into their mouths.

### Symptoms of choking

Sometimes people – especially children and older people – choke on food (or, in the case of young children, other objects they have put in their mouths). Unconsciousness and even death can occur if the air passages are blocked for more than a few minutes. In all cases, you should be ready to resuscitate the casualty if necessary.

The figure on page 364 shows the symptoms of choking.

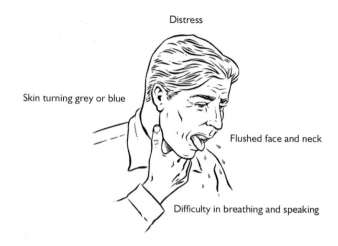

Distress

Skin turning grey or blue

Flushed face and neck

Difficulty in breathing and speaking

### *Choking in adults*

If the casualty is an adult and they are conscious:

- Tell them to cough
- Tell them to bend forwards
- Using the flat of your hand, give five firm slaps between the shoulder blades.

If this does not help:

- Stand behind the casualty
- Put your arms round the casualty so that one fist is below the ribcage
- Join your hands together and pull sharply inwards and upwards. This is an **abdominal thrust**
- Give up to five abdominal thrusts
- Give alternating back slaps and abdominal thrusts until the obstruction clears.

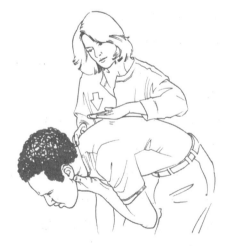

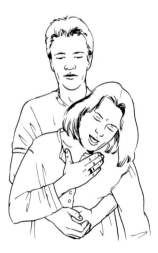

Never feel blindly down the person's throat, as you may push the obstruction further down. In all cases, be ready to resuscitate if necessary.

## Heart attack

A heart attack is caused by a blood clot blocking a coronary artery. The blood clot prevents blood reaching the heart.

### What are the signs and symptoms of a heart attack?

These are shown below.

*Signs of a heart attack*

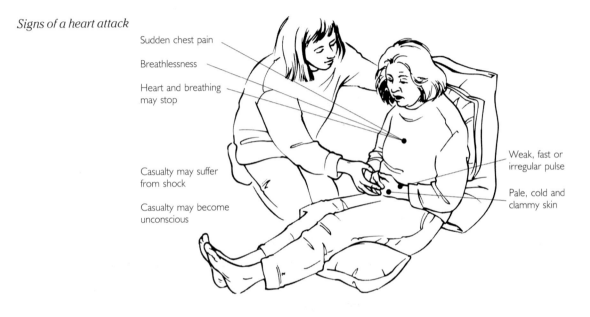

Sudden chest pain

Breathlessness

Heart and breathing may stop

Casualty may suffer from shock

Casualty may become unconscious

Weak, fast or irregular pulse

Pale, cold and clammy skin

### What can you do in a case of a heart attack?

Telephone for a doctor or ambulance.

Try not to move the casualty.

If the casualty is conscious:

1.  Place them in the W position (see figure on page 366).

2.  Loosen any tight clothing.

3.  Talk to the casualty and comfort them.

If the person is unconscious:

1.  Place them in the recovery position (see page 358).

2.  Get medical help as soon as possible.

3.  Check the casualty's pulse and breathing every 10 minutes.

4.  If heart and breathing stops, start resuscitation (see page 360).

*The W position*

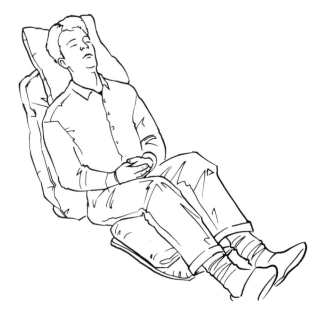

**Demonstrate and understand the correct first aid procedures when dealing with bleeding, including wounds where there is an embedded object**

### Bleeding

It is important to recognise the difference between a small wound that is bleeding a little and a serious wound from which blood flows or spurts out. The word **haemorrhage** is sometimes used to describe heavy bleeding.

Don't panic if you see blood, but you must consider your own safety. Avoid contact with blood and body fluids. Read and remember the following rules:

### *Dealing with blood and body fluids*

- Avoid contact with blood and body fluids
- Wear protective latex gloves when in contact with them
- Wash hands thoroughly in soap and water if you touch blood or body fluids
- Avoid contact with cuts and abrasions
- Cover open wounds with waterproof dressings
- Food handlers should use blue waterproof dressings.

### *Disinfection*

- Wear latex gloves and a plastic apron when mopping up
- Disinfect areas contaminated with blood and body fluids with a bleach solution

- Dispose of contaminated waste using the appropriate bags and containers.

### Did you know?

- The average adult has 6 litres of blood circulating in his/her body
- A healthy adult can donate half a litre of blood without any ill effect.

## External bleeding

This is usually quite obvious, although it can sometimes be hidden from view by the casualty's clothing. Blood flow can be anything from a slow trickle to a rhythmic spurt.

Types of wounds that can occur:

- Cut
- Bruise
- Laceration (torn flesh)
- Graze
- Puncture.

Apart from the actual presence of blood, there are other signs and symptoms that show that serious bleeding is taking place (see below).

*Signs of serious bleeding*

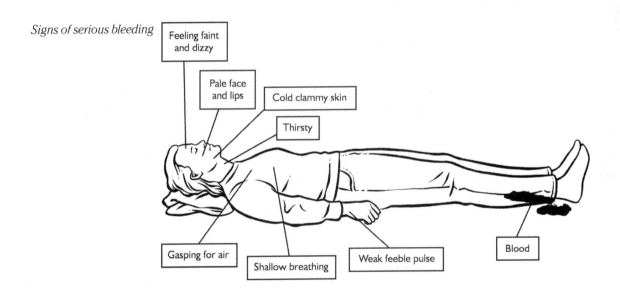

### What to do if someone is bleeding

- Get help if there is no sign of the bleeding lessening or if a lot of blood has already been lost
- If possible, wear disposable gloves
- Talk to the casualty
- Apply a dressing
- Apply pressure to the wound for up to 10 minutes
- Depending upon the site of the bleeding, lie or sit the casualty down

11

*Applying pressure and raising a bleeding leg*

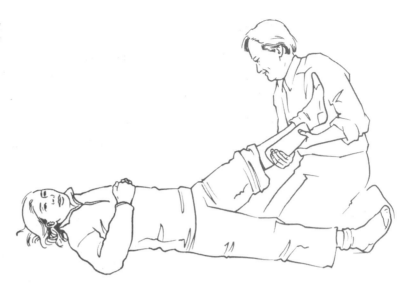

- If possible, raise the affected part to reduce the flow of blood (see above)
- Leave the original dressing in place, adding more dressings on top if necessary
- Treat for shock (see page 369)
- Get the casualty to hospital.

## Internal bleeding

Sometimes a casualty shows the symptoms of bleeding but no actual blood is visible. This could mean that there is bleeding inside the body. First aiders call this **internal bleeding**.

The figure below shows what to do if you suspect someone has internal bleeding.

*Internal bleeding: what to do*

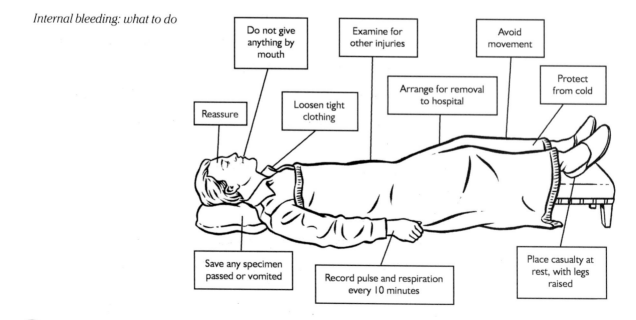

Do not give anything by mouth

Examine for other injuries

Avoid movement

Protect from cold

Reassure

Loosen tight clothing

Arrange for removal to hospital

Save any specimen passed or vomited

Record pulse and respiration every 10 minutes

Place casualty at rest, with legs raised

## Shock

Many people have heard of the word **shock**. In the medical sense, it means a serious state of collapse that may accompany injuries, especially where there is loss of blood.

Severe bleeding can cause shock.

A severely shocked casualty will have the symptoms shown in the figure below

*Symptoms of shock*

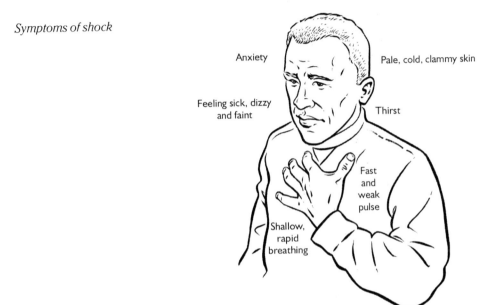

### What to do for a shocked casualty

- Put the casualty in a suitable position for the injury:
    - Minor injuries: sitting down
    - Unconscious casualties: recovery position as described on page 358
    - Chest injuries: sitting up and leaning to injured side
    - Heart conditions: 'W' position (see figure on page 366) or lying flat
    - Otherwise, lying flat with the feet raised if possible.
- If possible, deal with the cause
- Loosen any tight clothing, especially round the neck, chest and waist
- Reassure the casualty
- Get medical aid
- Observe the casualty carefully, monitoring pulse and breathing
- Never move the casualty unnecessarily, give food or drink or allow him/her to smoke.

# 12 Nutrition and cooking for health

## To complete this unit you will need to:

- Describe the dietary needs of different people in society
- Describe the functions and sources of nutrients and how they contribute to diet
- Demonstrate understanding of service users with specific dietary needs
- Plan meals for service users with different needs
- Produce a main meal to meet the requirements of a service user, evaluating its appropriateness for the service user
- Plan how to adapt recipes using different food sources for different service user groups.

**AO1   Describe the dietary needs of different people in society**

*The Health of the Nation*, a Government White Paper published in 1992 and then updated in 1993, set guidelines to improve the national diet. If the nation's diet improved then there would be fewer people who were obese or suffering from coronary heart disease. Targets set included reducing the number of heart disease and stroke deaths in the under-65s by at least 40%. This was to be achieved by the year 2000.

In a later report, *Our Healthier Nation* (1999), it was stated that, by the year 2005, the number of people aged 16–64 who were obese was to be reduced by 25% for men and 33% for women. Hopefully the amount of fat in the average diet would be reduced by 12% to approximately 30% of food energy.

The Ministry of Agriculture, Food and Fisheries (MAFF) produced a checklist for a balanced diet from which 'The Balance of Good Health' was produced in 1994. The following is the MAFF checklist:

- Enjoy your food
- Eat a variety of different foods
- Eat the right amount to stay at a healthy weight
- Eat plenty of foods rich in starch or fibre
- Don't eat too much fat
- Don't eat sugary food too often
- Look after the vitamins and minerals in your food
- If you drink alcohol, keep within sensible limits.

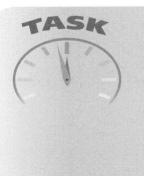

## TASK

### The Balance of Good Health

Divide your Health and Social Care group into three. Each group should choose a different promotion method to present MAFF's 'The Balance of Good Health'.

The following presentation methods could be used:

- Poster
- Video
- Dance
- Rap
- Role play
- Cartoon
- Story, etc.

'The Balance of Good Health' is based on five commonly accepted food groups. These are:

- Bread, other cereals and potatoes
- Fruit and vegetables
- Milk and dairy foods
- Meat, fish and other alternatives
- Fatty and sugary food.

Fortunately there is no need to carry round a book of nutrients. For most people it is sufficient to sort foods into different classes and eat samples from each class. This is the basis of the *Balance of Good Health National Food Guide*. In the Guide, foods are divided into five groups, as illustrated in the figure on page 378.

The Committee on Medical Aspects of Food Policy – COMA – produced a report entitled *Dietary Reference Values for Food Energy and Nutrients for the UK*. This was published in 1991, and updated dietary requirements.

Not everybody has the same nutritional needs. It very much depends on the person's age, gender, height and how active they are.

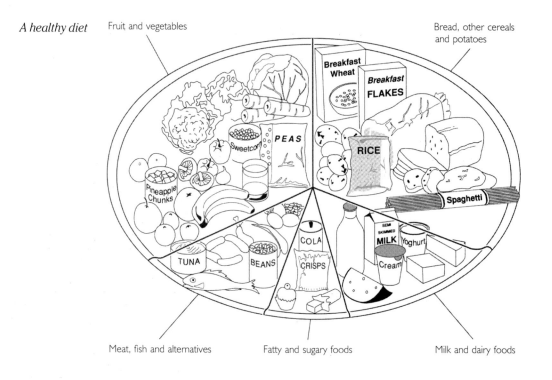

*A healthy diet*

Fruit and vegetables

Bread, other cereals and potatoes

Meat, fish and alternatives

Fatty and sugary foods

Milk and dairy foods

## TASK

### Nutritional needs

Would a 3-year-old girl have the same nutritional needs as a 15-year-old boy? If not, why not?

## Current dietary reference values

Dietary reference values have been estimated for groups of people with similar characteristics, such as age, sex and level of physical activity. Dietary reference values include reference nutrient intakes (RNIs), estimated average requirements (EARs) and lower reference nutrient intakes (LRNIs).

### Reference nutrient intake (RNI)

The RNI is the amount of a nutrient that would be enough for nearly everyone – in fact this level of intake is higher than most people need.

### Estimated average requirement (EAR)

The EAR is an estimate of the average need for food energy or a nutrient. This is the estimated average for a group of people and is not meant to be the recommended intake for an individual.

## Lower reference nutrient intake (LRNI)

The LRNI refers to the very small percentage of the population who have low needs.

*Table 12.1 Daily dietary recommendations*

| Energy and nutrients | Dietary recommendations |
|---|---|
| Energy | EARS for energy vary with age, sex and level of activity, e.g. |
| | Adult man     10,600 kilojoules (kJ) daily |
| | Adult woman    8,100kJ daily |
| Protein | RNI   55.5g   men |
| | 45g   women |
| Total fat | No more than 35% of food energy |
| | Saturates    No more than 11% of food energy |
| Carbohydrates | 50% of food energy |
| Dietary fibre | 12.24g for an adult |
| Vitamins | Each has own dietary recommendation |
| Minerals | Each has own dietary recommendation |

**Case Study**

Mr Ramsden, 63, in a wheelchair

Robert, 18 years old, cross country runner

Mrs Smith, 36, pregnant with third child

Lucy, 4 years old, just started school

Andrea, 17 years old, student

Mr Teasdale, 43, refuse collector

Mrs Edwards, 76, bowls champion

Mr Summerly, 57, retired gardener

*People have different energy needs at different times in their lives.*

*Consider the people listed above, and their lifestyles, and put them in order of their energy requirements, starting with the highest.*

## Factors influencing diet

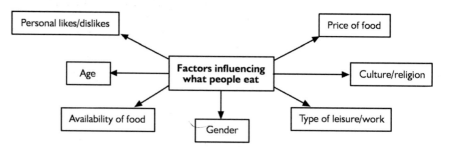

### Socioeconomic factors

These are very important, as the price of food has got to be taken into consideration. Most people have a strict budget that they wish or have to stick to. Availability of food will also affect price; for example, food items are normally more expensive when they are out of season.

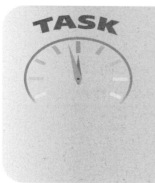

## TASK

### Budgeting for food

You are a 20-year-old single parent caring for a 2-year-old child.

Find out the current benefit allowance entitlement.

After you have paid all your bills, you have £35 left to spend on food.

Visit your local supermarket and work out what food you would buy to last the week.

## Nutritional requirements

### Older people

Although older people need less food for energy, their food should supply a range of nutrients. Healthy eating guidelines should be followed, with older people eating less fat and sugar and more foods rich in fibre.

- Protein should be easily digestible, as many older people have false teeth or few remaining teeth, and have difficulty chewing certain foods such as meat
- Vitamin C is necessary for general good health and gums, and to help the absorption of iron
- Iron to prevent anaemia
- Vitamin D to help with the absorption of calcium
- Calcium to prevent brittle bones and curved spine (osteoporosis)
- Cut down on salt to reduce risk of high blood pressure
- Fibre to prevent constipation.

Table 12.2 EARS for energy – older people

| Age | EAR (kJ daily) | | EAR (kcal daily) | |
|---|---|---|---|---|
| | Male | Female | Male | Female |
| 60–64 | 9,930 | 7,990 | 2,380 | 1,900 |
| 65–74 | 9,710 | 7,960 | 2,330 | 1,900 |
| 75+ | 8,770 | 7,610 | 2,100 | 1,810 |

There is good evidence that levels of calcium and vitamin D need to be increased to prevent or delay the process of calcium loss from bones. This particularly affects women after the menopause, but it also affects men.

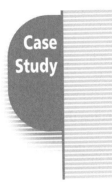

**Case Study**

Mr and Mrs Dawson are in their early seventies. Both are in good health and enjoy hill walking.

*Suggest a suitable menu for their meals for one day. Ensure that the foods you have chosen include the main nutrients necessary for older people: protein, vitamin C, iron, vitamin D, calcium and fibre.*

*In each dish, identify the main nutrient.*

### Adults

Throughout adulthood, differences in dietary requirements are largely related to physical activity and differences in size. If you carry out the calculations for different nutrient requirements per kilogram of body weight you will find that there is very little difference between men and women. The differences in the daily requirements are related to the fact that the average adult woman is smaller than the average adult man.

To a lesser extent, there are sex differences with regard to requirements for specific nutrients. The male hormone testosterone affects protein requirements and so men require slightly more than women for equivalent physically active lifestyles. Women have a greater requirement for iron.

Table 12.3 EARS for energy – younger adults

| Age | EAR (kJ daily) | | EAR (kcal daily) | |
|---|---|---|---|---|
| | Male | Female | Male | Female |
| 19–50 | 10,600 | 8,100 | 2,550 | 1,940 |
| 51–59 | 10,600 | 8,000 | 2,550 | 1,900 |

Adults have stopped growing and are usually less active than teenagers. They still need a well balanced diet with a good range of macro- and micronutrients.

### Sources of fat

Sources of fat in the diet can be from:

- Animals – most animal fats are solid at room temperature and contain a high proportion of saturated fats

- Plants – fats from plant sources are often liquid at room temperature and are usually called oils. These are normally found in seeds and fruits, such as corn, olives and avocados, and often contain a high proportion of unsaturated fats.

COMA recommends that we reduce the amount of fat we eat to no more than 35% of food energy, with not more than 11% coming from saturated fats.

**TASK**

## Composition of fats

Look in the chiller unit of your local big supermarket and note the selection of fats available, e.g.:

- Lurpak
- Kerrygold
- Clover
- Flora
- Utterly Butterly
- Bertolli
- Stork – block
- Trex
- St Ivel Mono
- St Ivel Gold
- Vitalite
- Benecol
- Dripping
- Baking margarine
- Pure with soya.

Draw up a table comparing their content of saturated, mono-unsaturated and polyunsaturated fats:

| Saturated fat | Mono-unsaturated fat | Polyunsaturated fat |
|---|---|---|
| Beef dripping | | |
| etc. | | |

## Dietary fibre

Dietary fibre is known as *non-starch polysaccharide* (NSP). It is derived from carbohydrate sources and is not digestible. As it cannot be digested, it passes through the gut, absorbing water and becoming bulkier. This is necessary for the digestive system to function properly – dietary fibre prevents constipation, bowel complaints and piles. Fibre also helps people reduce their weight, as it is very filling.

There are two types of dietary fibre – soluble and insoluble.

- Soluble fibre helps to slow down digestion of carbohydrates, thereby levelling out blood sugar levels and helping to prevent hunger
- Insoluble fibre goes through the body absorbing water and collecting waste materials, keeping faeces soft and regular.

COMA recommends that adults increase the amount of fibre to between 12 and 24 grams per day.

There is some evidence that soluble fibre found in things like oats may affect blood cholesterol levels and reduce the risk of heart attacks. However, we do not yet fully understand the link and how it might work.

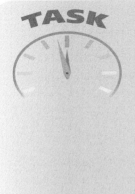

## TASK

## Composition of fats

Fibre is essential in a balanced diet. Compare the fibre content of the following foods:

- Minced beef
- Wholemeal bread
- White sliced bread
- Wholemeal pasta
- Basmati rice
- Lentil soup
- Milk chocolate

- Baked beans
- Tinned peaches
- Dried prunes
- Orange juice
- Brown rice
- Eggs
- Tofu.

### Water

This is not usually regarded as a food, but it is important in the diet. Every part and function of the body depends on water and it is being lost continuously through the skin, lungs, kidneys and bowels. This water must be replaced and is obtained from the liquids that we drink and the food that we eat.

## Nutritional deficiencies

Everyone has different nutritional needs, and some people can cope with nutritional deficiencies better than others. It was noticed that prisoners of war who were given exactly the same diet suffered a range of effects, from being hardly affected (apart from weight loss) to blindness and death.

The body is able to adapt to reduced food intake, but too little food over a period of time can lead to ill-health through under-nutrition. In extreme cases, as in developing countries of the world, starvation causes stunting of physical and mental development, and wasting. Diseases such as scurvy and some forms of anaemia are caused by a deficiency (shortage) of certain nutrients or by the body's inability to absorb them.

12

In the UK, we may not necessarily have the problem of starvation, but excessive amounts of food can also cause malnutrition (literally, 'bad eating'), which may lead to conditions of ill-health such as obesity, heart disease or high blood pressure. Too much sugar, for example, may cause tooth decay. In poor countries, diets are often low in fat, while in the West we are advised to reduce our fat intake to prevent heart disease. Adults and children over 5 years are recommended to avoid taking in more than one-third of their total energy or calorie intake in the form of fat.

It is useful to check labels on products and prepared foods just to see the amount of fat or sugar in the product. The greatest amount is listed first. There has been some publicity (and disagreement) about certain fats being connected with particular diseases. It is thought that high intakes of saturated fats (lard, suet, cocoa butter) may increase the cholesterol level in some individuals and so increase the risk of heart disease.

Some nutrients are necessary for good health. The possible effects of deficiencies of these nutrients are mentioned below. Don't forget that people have differing needs.

## Carbohydrate deficiency

If a person's carbohydrate intake is too low, their protein intake has to be used for energy and so the 'growth and repair' function of the protein has less effect.

## Mineral deficiency

### Iron

Deficiency of iron can result in anaemia (a decrease in the ability of the blood to carry oxygen to the body's cells). A person with anaemia may feel tired and lethargic and be pale. Anaemia can also arise from a shortage of folic acid and vitamin $B_{12}$. The absorption of iron from food is generally low, but it is increased when the body's stores are low, as during menstruation.

### Calcium

Calcium is the most abundant mineral in the body. Too little calcium in young children may result in stunted growth and rickets (a condition where the bones develop badly and the legs are bowed). The condition is rarely seen in the UK today. Among elderly people, the condition may show as osteomalacia. The main cause of such conditions is lack of vitamin D, which assists the absorption of calcium.

### Phosphorus

Phosphorus is found in many foods and it is difficult to have too little in the diet. If too much phosphorus is taken in the first few days of life, however, this may produce low levels of calcium in the blood and muscular spasms.

Phosphorus is found in cows' milk and that is why babies must only have 'modified' milk, special baby milk or breast milk.

### Sodium

Sodium and water requirements are closely linked. Too little sodium may result in muscle cramps. Salt is present naturally in foods and many prepared foods have a high salt content (check the labels). Habitual high salt intake is associated with high blood pressure. Babies under 1 year old and people with kidney complaints or water retention problems cannot tolerate a high salt intake.

### Potassium

Losses of potassium may be large if laxatives or diuretics (medication to reduce water retention) are used or if the carbohydrate intake level is so low that protein is used for energy. In extreme cases, deficiency of potassium can result in heart failure.

### Fluorine

Fluorine is found in tea, seafood, toothpaste and water. The fluorine or fluoride level in tap water varies in different parts of the country. Fluoride can help to prevent tooth decay. Take care, however, because an excess of fluoride can cause the teeth to become mottled.

### Iodine

A shortage of iodine causes the thyroid gland to swell – this condition is known as goitre.

### Zinc

If a diet is too high in fibre, the zinc in food may not be absorbed and this may affect growth and repair.

More knowledge is needed about the trace elements (fluorine, iodine and zinc). The full effects of deficiencies of them aren't fully understood; neither is it known how one may affect another.

### *Vitamin deficiency*

In general terms, a shortage of vitamins can lead to a reduced resistance to disease and feeling unwell. An excess of certain vitamins can also be harmful. The more specific deficiencies are:

- Vitamin A – poor vision and, in extreme cases, blindness; however, an excess of vitamin A is poisonous.
- Vitamin $B_1$ (thiamine) – depression, tiredness and, in cases of severe lack, diseases of the nervous system; also beriberi in rice-eating communities.

- Vitamin B$_2$ (riboflavin) – rarely deficient; occasionally deficiency causes sores in the mouth. Can be destroyed by sunlight, so avoid leaving milk on a sunny doorstep.

- Nicotinic acid (niacin) – in famine areas this causes pellagra, a condition where the skin becomes dark and scaly when exposed to light.

- Vitamin C – bleeding from small blood vessels and gums; wounds heal more slowly. Prolonged lack causes scurvy. There is no scientific evidence that a lack of vitamin C means more colds.

- Vitamin D – rickets and osteoporosis (see Calcium deficiency, above).

## AO3 Demonstrate understanding of service users with specific dietary needs

Not everyone is free to eat the foods they would like to. Some people have special dietary requirements.

### Coeliac disease

Coeliac disease is the result of an allergic reaction to gluten. Gluten is a protein found in wheat, oats, barley and rye. With coeliac disease, the lining of the small intestine is hypersensitive to gluten and this prevents nutrients from being properly absorbed, so weight loss occurs. If a child has coeliac disease, and it is undetected, the child's growth could be permanently stunted, as the child will suffer from malnutrition.

#### Dietary requirements for coeliac disease

- All foods containing gluten, e.g. cakes, breads, biscuits, pastries, pasta and cereals, must be cut from the diet. Nothing made from or containing wheat, oats, barley or rye should be eaten.

- Always check food labels carefully as many unexpected foods, such as non-dairy ice cream, cocoa powder and table sauces, contain gluten.

- Many food products have 'gluten-free' on the label.

*Look out for the gluten-free symbol on food packaging*

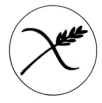

### Irritable bowel syndrome

The cause of irritable bowel is not fully understood but it is thought that anxiety or emotional stress can contribute to this condition.

## Cause and effects of irritable bowel syndrome

Many people's symptoms are so mild that they don't bother go to their GP. Other people can have symptoms that are more troublesome, especially abdominal cramps, bloating and diarrhoea.

The most common symptom is abdominal pain, which some people describe as aching or colicky. The pain may be mild or severe, and may be made either better or worse by opening the bowels, passing wind or eating. Pain may recur at a particular time of day, often in the evening.

People with this condition often feel an urgent need to open their bowels, especially after breakfast. The stools may vary in consistency from hard and pellet-like to loose and watery, or just small amounts of mucus. Afterwards, there may be a sense that the bowels have not been completely emptied.

Other symptoms include a bloated abdomen, excess wind, nausea, vomiting and indigestion. Some people also experience a sense of fullness. If the main symptom is diarrhoea, food passes through the digestive system faster than usual.

The exact cause of irritable bowel is not known. It is termed a functional disorder, which means that the way the bowel works is affected, but no physical abnormalities that might explain the symptoms have been found.

Symptoms are thought to be caused by muscle contractions in the bowel wall. The contractions may be most troublesome after food and in stressful situations. Intolerance of specific foods (such as tea, coffee and dairy products) may trigger the symptoms.

### *Dietary requirements for irritable bowel syndrome*

It is recommended that the person follows a high fibre diet. Wholemeal flour should be used in bread, cakes, biscuits, and pastries. A diet rich in fruits and vegetables will also be beneficial. Wholegrain breakfast cereals, nuts, seeds, peas, beans and lentils are all good sources of fibre.

## Diets for people with diabetes

Diabetes is a disorder of the body's internal control of blood glucose levels. Insulin is produced by the pancreas and the mechanism is controlled by the level of blood glucose. Diabetics either produce:

- No insulin or
- Too little insulin.

### *Diabetics who produce no insulin*

People with this form of diabetes usually have to inject themselves with a mixture of slow-acting and fast-acting insulin designed to match their sugar intake and needs. The aim in controlling diabetes is to keep blood sugar levels within acceptable norms and as steady as possible.

The skill in planning a diet for a diabetic is to provide the carbohydrate in forms that allow sugar to pass into the bloodstream in a way that mirrors the available insulin. The diabetic person has to space out meals and eat carbohydrate between meals to match the energy requirements. This means that a diabetic planning to undertake vigorous exercise may prepare by eating a sweet biscuit to balance the sugar required for the exercise.

A high-fibre diet is useful for insulin-injecting diabetics as it helps reduce the swings in blood sugar levels and balances the fast- and slow-acting insulin that is injected.

### Diabetics who produce some insulin

These people need to try to balance their carbohydrate (starches and sugars) intake with the amount of insulin produced. One important way of doing this is to have a diet that is high in fibre. This has the effect of slowing the digestion of starches and so releasing sugars at a reasonably steady rate. These are absorbed from the intestines into the bloodstream at a similar steady rate. The limited amount of insulin produced is sufficient to cope with this steady intake of sugar. Without the fibre the digested sugars would be absorbed rapidly and would overwhelm the limited supply of insulin.

Key things to monitor in diets for diabetics are:

- Sugar content (glucose and sucrose)
- Complex carbohydrates (starches and fibre).

## Food intolerance

### Lactose intolerance – causes and effects

Lactose intolerance is the inability to digest significant amounts of lactose, the predominant sugar of milk. This inability results from a shortage of the enzyme lactase, which is normally produced by the cells that line the small intestine. Lactase breaks down milk sugar into simpler forms that can then be absorbed into the bloodstream. When there is not enough lactase to digest the amount of lactose consumed, the results, although not usually dangerous, may be very distressing. While not all persons deficient in lactase have symptoms, those who do are considered to be lactose intolerant.

Some causes of lactose intolerance are well known. For instance, certain digestive diseases and injuries to the small intestine can reduce the amount of enzymes produced. In rare cases, children are born without the ability to produce lactase. For most people, though, lactase deficiency is a condition that develops naturally over time.

Common symptoms include nausea, cramps, bloating, gas, and diarrhoea, which begin about 30 minutes to 2 hours after eating or drinking foods containing lactose. The severity of symptoms varies depending on the amount of lactose each individual can tolerate.

Lactose intolerance does not pose a serious threat to good health. People who have trouble digesting lactose can learn which dairy products and other foods they can eat without discomfort and which ones they should avoid. Many will be able to enjoy milk, ice cream, and other such products if they take them in small amounts or eat other food at the same time. Others can use lactase liquid or tablets to help digest the lactose. Even older women at risk of osteoporosis and growing children who must avoid milk and foods made with milk can meet most of their special dietary needs by eating greens, fish, and other calcium-rich foods that are free of lactose.

## Food allergies

As allergies can be life threatening it is a good idea to ask service users if they have any known allergy. Common allergies are to peanuts, shellfish, eggs, soya and certain colourings and preservatives. If the allergy is known about, it is then easy to avoid it.

## AO4    Plan meals for service users with different needs

### Reference nutrient intakes

Table 12.6 shows some daily requirements for different groups of people – the reference nutrient intakes. You will see that carbohydrate is not included (other than fibre). This is because it is part of the energy intake and the amount required varies according to the amount of fat and excess protein in the diet. Throughout this unit we will not expect you to calculate carbohydrate intake unless you choose to find information for a diabetic diet.

### Food tables

To know what nutrients different foods contain, you can use food tables that give the composition of foods per 100g. You may also be able to use one of the many computer programs that help you to analyse your diet. However, the tables do not always give details of all possible foods.

### Benefits of a balanced diet

- By matching your diet to your needs, you give your body the opportunity to function at its most efficient. In such a situation you are also more likely to be physically fit. This does not mean that you are athletic. It means that your heart, lungs and the rest of your body are in balance and little stress is being caused to any part.

Table 12.6   *Reference nutrient intakes of selected nutrients, per day*

| Age range | Vitamin B6 (mg) | Folic acid (mg) | Protein (g) | Vitamin C (mg) | Calcium (mg) | Iron (mg) | Zinc (mg) | Vitamin A (mg) | Thiamine (mg) |
|---|---|---|---|---|---|---|---|---|---|
| 0–3 months (formula-fed) | 0.2 | 50 | 12.5 | 25 | 525 | 1.7 | 4.0 | 350 | 0.2 |
| 4–6 months | 0.2 | 50 | 12.7 | 25 | 525 | 4.3 | 4.0 | 350 | 0.2 |
| 7–9 months | 0.3 | 50 | 13.7 | 25 | 525 | 7.8 | 5.0 | 350 | 0.2 |
| 10–12 months | 0.4 | 50 | 14.9 | 25 | 525 | 7.8 | 5.0 | 350 | 0.3 |
| 1–3 years | 0.7 | 70 | 14.5 | 30 | 350 | 6.9 | 5.0 | 400 | 0.5 |
| 4–6 years | 0.9 | 100 | 19.7 | 30 | 450 | 6.1 | 6.5 | 500 | 0.7 |
| 7–10 years | 1.0 | 150 | 28.3 | 30 | 550 | 8.7 | 5.0 | 500 | 0.7 |
| **Males** | | | | | | | | | |
| 11–14 years | 1.2 | 200 | 42.1 | 35 | 1,000 | 11.3 | 9.0 | 600 | 0.9 |
| 15–18 years | 1.5 | 200 | 55.2 | 40 | 1,000 | 11.3 | 9.5 | 700 | 1.1 |
| 19–50 years | 1.4 | 200 | 55.5 | 40 | 700 | 8.7 | 9.5 | 700 | 1.0 |
| 50+ years | 1.4 | 200 | 53.3 | 40 | 700 | 8.7 | 9.5 | 700 | 0.9 |
| **Females** | | | | | | | | | |
| 11–14 years | 1.0 | 200 | 41.2 | 35 | 800 | 14.8 | 9.0 | 600 | 0.7 |
| 15–18 years | 1.2 | 200 | 45.0 | 40 | 800 | 14.8 | 7.0 | 600 | 0.8 |
| 19–50 years | 1.2 | 200 | 45.0 | 40 | 700 | 14.8 | 7.0 | 600 | 0.8 |
| 50+ years | 1.2 | 200 | 46.5 | 40 | 700 | 8.7 | 7.0 | 600 | 0.8 |
| Pregnant* | – | +100 | +6.0 | +10 | – | – | – | +100 | +0.1 |
| Lactating* – 4 months | +11.0 | +550 | – | +6.0 | +350 | +0.2 | – | +60 | +30 |
| Over 4 months | +8.0 | +550 | – | +2.5 | +350 | +0.2 | – | +60 | +30 |

* For pregnant and lactating women the figures given are to be added to the amount for the woman's age range.
Source: Table 25 from MAFF, *Manual of nutrition* (HMSO, 1995)

- Monitoring and maintaining a balanced diet means that your weight should be correct for your height. This again means that your muscles and skeleton are in balance and are not being damaged by too much weight.

- A balanced diet can help prevent disease. Clearly you will not suffer any deficiency diseases or diseases of excess. General health and resistance to infection is also improved. This is because a balanced diet assists all the body systems to be in balance. This includes those involved in preventing and fighting disease.

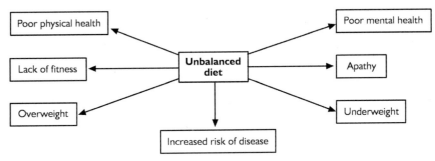

## Factors influencing dietary patterns

We all have different likes and dislikes in terms of food. We also all have different lifestyles. What you eat and when you eat is determined by a variety of things. These include the factors listed in the figure below.

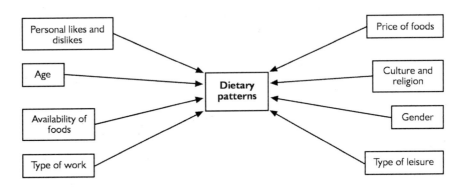

## Eating patterns

The pattern of meals for very young babies involves small intakes of food about every four hours. This pattern has evolved to provide the required nutrients without putting a great strain on the digestive system. It is thought that early people had a feeding pattern of frequent small meals with occasional large ones. This reflected the hunter–gatherer lifestyle.

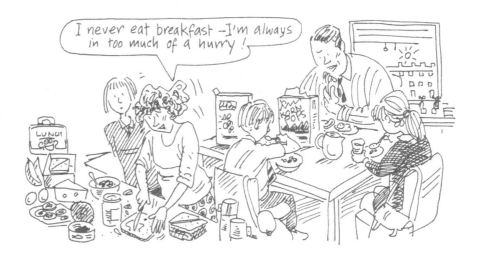

summer. Now it is possible to obtain most foods at any time of the year. However, the fact that the foods are in the shops does not mean that everyone can have them. Even though they are available, strawberries are very expensive at Christmas!

When planning a diet it is better to use foods that are in season, for two reasons:

- If they are in season, they cost less than out of season
- They may have a greater nutritional content because they are fresher. Nutrients such as vitamins may be lost as a result of storage while foods are transported across the world.

The latter can be an important factor in considering different foods. For example, potatoes are a source of vitamin C. Freshly dug potatoes have a higher vitamin C content than those that have been stored. As freshly dug potatoes are not available through the winter they cannot be seen as an important source of vitamin C.

Similar comments can be made about many fresh vegetables compared with those that have been tinned. It is important to note that the word 'fresh' is open to interpretation and to remember that many 'fresh' foods lose important nutrients if they are stored incorrectly for even a short period.

### Cost of food

As we have already indicated, the cost of food can have seasonal variations. More important here is a person's ability to buy the right food to produce a balanced diet. People living on low incomes or benefits may struggle to provide a balanced diet from the available income. There are regular articles in the press from people suggesting that it is possible to provide a balanced diet on a low income. This may be true, but the choice of foods becomes limited and the diet, while nutritious, could become boring and monotonous.

## Service users

Refer back to A01 for information on special dietary requirements.

### Children

- Children should be encouraged to eat a wide variety of foods
- Food should be served in small portions, as they have small appetites
- Food should be easy for children to manage, e.g. if necessary cut up into manageable-sized bites
- Make food attractive
- Do not give children fried, greasy or spicy foods, which they may find difficult to digest.

### Adults

Refer to the RNI chart for adults. Are there any special requirements, e.g. is the person trying to lose weight? Do they have any allergies? Likes/dislikes?

### Older people

- Remember to choose easily digested protein foods
- Avoid too many fried or spicy foods, which could cause indigestion
- Appetites are reduced, so serve smaller portions.

### Vegetarians

- What type of vegetarian will you be catering for?
- Remember to replace animal protein with good vegetable sources, such as peas, beans, lentils, etc.

Remember that the main meal, whether eaten at mid-day or in the evening, must contain a large percentage of the nutrients which the body will need throughout the day.

## AO5 Produce a main meal to meet the requirements of a service user, evaluating its appropriateness for the service user

Here are some examples of meals suitable for different service users. Refer to AO3 for guidelines.

### Children – main meal

Fish in butter sauce

Mashed potato

Carrots

Apple crumble

Custard

### Adults – Main Meal

Chicken casserole

Jacket potato

Broccoli

Fresh fruit salad

Yoghurt

### Older adults – main meal

Liver and onion

Boiled potato

Cabbage

Rice pudding

### Vegetarian (specify type)

Vegetable lasagne

Salad

Pineapple upside-down pudding

Custard

### Special dietary needs (e.g. irritable bowel) – main meal

Chilli con carne

Brown rice

Dried apricot crumble (made with wholemeal flour)

Custard

After you have chosen your meal, check the dietary reference values using a nutritional analysis programme such as 'Nutrients'. Did your chosen meal provide the correct amount of necessary nutrients? Did you have problems buying any of the ingredients? Was it difficult to make? Did it look appetising? Did it taste nice?

Would you advise this meal as a good choice for your service user? If not, why not?

 ## AO6 Plan how to adapt recipes using different food sources for different service user groups

Vegetarians can replace meat as the main ingredient in a dish by using textured vegetable proteins (TVP), Quorn or tofu. TVP and tofu are both products of soya beans, while Quorn is made from a fungus and can be bought in fillets, in pieces or minced.

Textured vegetable protein can be used to replace minced meat in most recipes, e.g. lasagne, cottage pie, pasties, burgers, sausages, curries and spaghetti bolognese.

Tofu can be used for savoury or sweet dishes, e.g. stir fries, sweet and sour dishes, curries, burgers, casseroles, kebabs, ice cream and fruit fools.

Quorn, too, can be used in curries, sweet and sour dishes and casseroles.

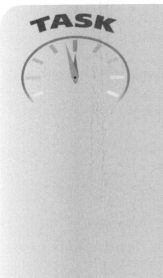

## Recipes using novel proteins

Choose a dish that can be made from a novel food as well as a traditional protein food (e.g. cottage pie). Cook both and compare the following:

- Cost of ingredients
- Ease of purchase of ingredients
- Storage of ingredients
- Preparation of meat/novel protein
- Length of time to cook
- Appearance
- Taste.

Could you tell the difference? Which did you prefer? Why?

Develop recipes to increase the amount of dietary fibre (NSP) and change the type of fat. Table 12.7 shows some possibilities.

*Table 12.7 Increasing the amount of dietary fibre in recipes and changing the type of fat*

| Food | Adaptation |
|---|---|
| White flour | Wholemeal varieties |
| Butter | Vegetable fats (polyunsaturated) <br> Low fat spreads |
| Whole milk | Skimmed/semi-skimmed |
| Cheese | Reduced fat varieties <br> Use well-flavoured cheeses, e.g. use 50g of Parmesan rather than 100g of Cheshire |
| Cream | Low fat cream <br> Fromage frais <br> Quark <br> Greek yoghurt |

The following recipes have been adapted to add fibre and reduce fat:

### Lasagne

| **Traditional** | **Adapted** |
|---|---|
| 175g lasagne | 175g *wholemeal* lasagne |
| **Cheese sauce** | |
| 375ml milk | 375ml *semi-skimmed* milk |
| 25g margarine | – |
| 25g plain flour | 25g cornflour |

½ level teaspoon mustard          ½ level teaspoon mustard
100g cheese                       50g *mature* cheese
**Meat sauce**
500g minced beef                  500g lean, healthy-eating minced steak
1 tablespoon oil                  –
1 small can tomatoes              1 small can tomatoes
1 onion                           1 onion
pinch mixed herbs                 pinch mixed herbs

Add fibre:
Wholemeal lasagne has been used to add fibre.

Cut down on fat:
In the white sauce, margarine and flour have been missed out and replaced with cornflour
The amount of cheese has been halved by using stronger-flavoured cheese
Full-fat milk has been replaced by semi-skimmed
Lean mince has been used, which will be dry-fried without oil.

**Apple crumble**

| Traditional | Adapted |
|---|---|
| 150g white flour | 150g *wholemeal* flour |
| 75g hard margarine | 75g *polyunsaturated* fat |
| 75g sugar | 75g sugar |
| 500g apple, peeled and sliced | 500g apple, cored and sliced |
| 75g sugar | 50g sugar |
| | ½ teaspoon cinnamon |

Wholemeal flour adds fibre to crumble topping
Apples have skin left on for extra fibre
Polyunsaturated fat has been substituted for hard margarine
The amount of sugar for sweetening apples has been reduced, and cinnamon has been added for extra flavour.

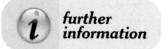

*further information*

Barker C et al (1999) *GCSE Design and Technology Food Technology.* Causeway Press Ltd

Clarke L (2002) *Health and Social Care GCSE.* Nelson Thornes, Cheltenham

Fox B and Cameron A (1995) *Food Science, Nutrition and Health.* Hodder & Stoughton, London

McCance RA and Widdowson EM (2001) *The Composition of Foods*, 6th edn. Royal Society of Chemistry, Cambridge

McGrath H (1994) *All About Food.* Oxford University Press, Oxford

www.allergyuk.org – Food allergy

www.bbc.co.uk/health/heart – BBC online health

www.bhf.org.uk – British Heart Foundation

www.coeliac.co.uk – Coeliac UK

www.diabetes.org.uk – Diabetes

www.food.gov.uk – Food Standards Publications

www.foodstandards.gov.uk – Food Standards Agency

www.heartstats.org – Statistics on Heart Disease

www.nutrition.org.uk – British Nutrition Foundation

www.ohn.gov.uk – Our Healthier Nation

www.sportex.net – Sport Ex Health

www.whi.org.uk – Walking for Health

## Summary

- Different people in society have different dietary requirements. For example, as people reach old age they should generally eat less fat and sugar and small children need high levels of calcium and protein for bone development and general growth and repair.

- Nutrients all have their specific functions and sources. For example, carbohydrates are an important source of energy and can be found in bread, potatoes and rice (starches) and jams, biscuits and chocolate (sugars).

- Specific dietary needs affect what foods service users can eat. For example, people with diabetes need to monitor the sugar content of the food they consume.

- When planning a meal for a service user, it must contain the correct balance of nutrients for their specific needs and be of an appropriate size.

- Adapting recipes to cater for specific dietary needs is a way of ensuring variety and nutrition for service users. For example, vegetarians can replace meat with textured vegetable protein as the main ingredient of a dish.

# 13 Creative activities with individuals in care settings

## To complete this unit you will need to:

- Recognise the needs of service users when planning creative activities, explaining the benefits of creative activities
- Describe a range of different types of creative activities available to service users and their purpose
- Describe the planning process for a creative activity and the importance of the stages within the programme planning
- Plan and carry out a creative activity for an individual
- Evaluate the creative activity
- Describe how the activity could be adapted for a service user with different needs.

 **AO1** Recognise the needs of service users when planning creative activities, explaining the benefits of creative activities

We are all creative beings: we express our creativity in the choices we make in our everyday lives; the clothes we wear, the colours we like, the way we decorate our homes and design our gardens, the music we listen to and the songs we sing.

The world of nature is also filled with wonderful creative designs such as the shape of a single snowflake, the colour and pattern of a leaf or the brilliant blues of a peacock's feather.

Evidence of creativity is all around us, making our lives richer, brighter, more imaginative and more meaningful.

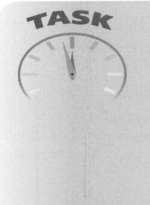

## TASK

### How creative are you?

- Have you ever designed and made a greetings card, e.g. Christmas card, valentine?
- Have you ever cooked and presented a meal?
- Do you have any posters on your bedroom wall at home?
- When was the last time you danced to a tape or video at home?

Working in small groups, discuss how creative you are, your interests and your skills.

If you had to choose a creative activity, which one would you choose and why?

We will all give different answers but we are all creative in our own different ways.

These are just a few examples and you will be able to think of many more. All these creative activities help to express and define who we are and what makes us special and unique.

Our imagination is without limit. By using our creative skills and resources available we can bring our thoughts and feelings to life and share them with other people.

Some people may need assistance and encouragement to express their imaginative ideas fully and confidently. Service users may have a range of needs, including:

- Reduced physical ability
- Mental health needs
- Learning disability
- Behavioural conditions
- People who need to return to the community after a period of rehabilitation
- Sensory impairment
- Special needs.

Everyone, in all care settings, should be given the opportunity to develop their creative skills and to express their creativity in their own way. Facilities, support and professional help should be available to them. Some voluntary organisations such as Age Concern, Scope and the Royal National Institute for the Blind actively promote this kind of service in care settings and often visit settings to carry out creative programmes.

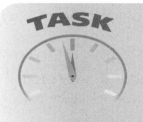

## Creative activities of voluntary organisations

Contact and arrange to visit a voluntary organisation in your area, for example, Alzheimer's Society, Mind, Age Concern.

Find out about the clients they work with, what are their needs?

Visit websites to find out information about client needs, e.g. www.ageconcern.org.uk, www.scope.org.uk, www.rnid.org.uk (the Royal National Institute for Deaf People), www.rnib.org.uk (the Royal National Institute of the Blind).

In each case, investigate how the organisation you have looked at provides opportunities for their clients to meet their creative needs.

Care users for this unit include:

- Children
- Adults in care settings
- Older people in care settings.

Care settings for this unit include:

- Nurseries
- Early years centres
- Special needs schools
- Residential care centres for young people with physical disabilities or learning difficulties
- Care homes for older people
- Sheltered accommodation
- Supported independent living for people with special needs
- Day centres
- Hospices.

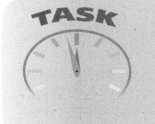

## Creative activities in care settings

In small groups, arrange a visit to one of the above care settings that provides creative activities for service users.

Participate in or observe the creative activities on offer.

## Needs of children, adults and older people in care settings

### Special needs

Special needs in children and young adults can range from being 'gifted and talented' to needing learning support. An assessment of needs may include the need for:

- Physical stimulation, e.g. kinetic learning, where the child is physically involved and active in the learning and creative process
- Intellectually challenging material to stimulate brain activity
- Emotional support and encouragement.

### Learning difficulties

This can include a range of disorders and conditions. Elderly people in care homes may have learning difficulties as a result of a stroke. Children may have learning difficulties as a result of a recognised condition such as dyspraxia or attention deficit hyperactivity disorder (ADHD), sometimes known as Attention Deficit Disorder (ADD). An assessment of needs may include some of the following:

- The need for concentration levels to be improved
- Opportunity for physical co-ordination
- Increasing confidence and building up self-esteem
- Developing intellectual skills.

### Physical disabilities

Physical disabilities affect the body. Disabilities may be caused by many conditions, including spina bifida, cerebral palsy, muscular dystrophy, Parkinson's disease and multiple sclerosis.

Needs to be promoted can include:

- Gross and fine motor skills
- Physical co-ordination
- Confidence in physical ability
- Integrating with others
- Building up muscle tone and strength, stamina and suppleness
- Social integration.

Some service users may suffer from arthritis and have a limited range of movement. It is important to offer support so that service users can join in any creative activities. There is sometimes a tendency for activities to be organised for people with similar disabilities. These can be very useful as self help groups but they tend to limit contact with others. Care workers must also assess the service users need for social integration with other groups of people.

### Sensory impairment

This is where the senses of sight, touch, hearing and smell are limited or damaged in some way. The most common types of impairment are hearing and sight loss. Carers need to be aware of such impairments when planning creative activities. Very often, if one sense is impaired another sense will become more highly developed to compensate for the loss. So, for example, someone who is visually impaired may have especially good hearing.

Needs to be promoted can include:

- A sensory environment, where materials can be touched and explored using the functioning senses safely
- A safe environment
- A full range of activities available, such as sculpting for the visually impaired
- Socialising with others in joint, collaborative activities.

### Behavioural conditions

Some syndromes can affect the behaviour patterns of people. They can behave without an awareness of socially acceptable boundaries; their behaviour can be compulsive and repetitive (ritualised behaviour). Some people suffering from trauma, shock and distress can also adopt behavioural patterns that can be very different from normal. The behaviour can also be very challenging.

Creative activities could address the need to:

- Build up self esteem, emotional well being and stability
- Develop an understanding of self and awareness of the feelings of others
- Develop social skills
- Develop a sense of enjoyment and a positive outlook.

### Mental health

Nearly one in twenty people experience some kind of mental health problem in their lifetime. These can include depression, compulsive obsessive disorders and schizophrenia. Schizophrenia most commonly occurs in young men and is evident when the sufferer feels disconnected from reality. This condition can be controlled by medication. In the stressful world we live in, children can have mental health problems and this is becoming more recognised. Anorexia and bulimia have also been connected to mental health problems.

Creative activities could address the need to:

- Socially interact and communicate with others
- Express emotions

- Build a strong, robust self image
- Provide intellectual understanding of themselves and their relation to the world around them.

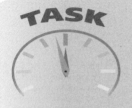

## Special needs

What do you understand about the following:

- ADHD (ADD)
- Dyspraxia
- Anorexia
- Bulimia
- Cerebral palsy
- Spina bifida
- Down's syndrome.

Some websites that may be useful are listed at the end of this unit.

You could also invite professionals from the organisation into school/ college. Their telephone numbers will be listed in your local yellow pages.

### Skills needed to return to the community

There are many short term rehabilitation programmes. These can include the care user who is in short-term stay in residential care, after an operation for example. It can also involve the support of people who are being rehabilitated back into the community, perhaps after being homeless, living rough or being drug-dependent. There are schemes to help people acquire the skills to adapt to living in the community and care workers whose job it is to assist with daily living needs. The care worker needs to:

- Boost the service user's self esteem
- Improve physical, practical skills such as cooking, decorating and shopping
- Provide opportunities for social networking within which experiences can be shared and new friendships formed
- Encourage intellectual and emotional development such as keeping a diary, writing down personal feelings. This is both creative and therapeutic.

## Benefits of creative activities

Creative activities are important for health and well-being. You will already be familiar with the idea of keeping fit to maintain health, but being involved in creative activities helps to maintain more than just physical health. The role of creative activities in maintaining and promoting intellectual, physical, social and emotional development is also important.

*Benefits of creative activity*

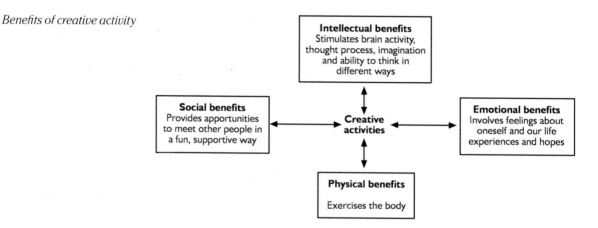

Some physical benefits from creative activities are to do with the development of motor skills. This can be particularly important when working with young children who, because of their age, are still at an early developmental stage and need opportunities to develop gross motor skills (refer back to Unit 7 to check developmental milestones). It can also be very important when working with people with physical disabilities who can experience difficulties with limb and hand movements. Some elderly service users may suffer from arthritis or have had a stroke, and their mobility may be affected as a result. Taking part in creative activities can help to exercise the affected areas and help to restore function and confidence.

*Creative activities encourage the use of both gross and fine motor skills*

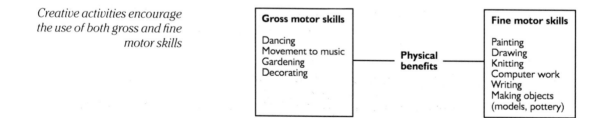

It is important to activate the brain and keep mentally alert throughout all stages of our lives. The intellectual benefits of creative activities can be stimulating, satisfying and enjoyable. Life-long learning is now recognised as essential to our development, well-being and sense of being valued.

### Social and emotional benefits from creative activities

People are naturally social beings and have a fundamental need for social contact and the opportunity to form relationships. As we develop we acquire social skills. Young children, for example, can appear to be very selfish. They do not know how to share but gradually learn to adapt to social situations, learning social skills and forming friends as they develop. An important part of a teenager's life is the opportunity for social networking and this can be a time of social explosion, during which they explore new situations and friendship groups. For older people the issue of social contact can be equally important; they may feel isolated and cut off from their friends, or they may be bereaved. Bringing people together to explore their creative skills in a social situation can be rewarding for both the service user and the care worker.

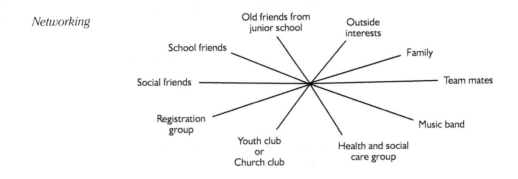

*Networking*

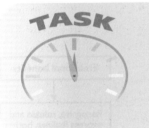

## Networking

Using the headings in the figure above as a guideline, write down all the people you know in each group.

Creative activities can also bring emotional benefits. It is probably impossible to extricate the emotions from creative activities. What we make and create will have our emotional fingerprints upon it.

## Benefits of creative activities

Read through the following statements. Decide which benefits are being gained from the activity: physical (P), intellectual (I), emotional (E) or social (S). Tick the appropriate boxes.

P    I    E    S

'I can't wait for Friday nights when I go out dancing. I feel so alive when I'm dancing, so connected, you know what I mean?' – (teenage girl)

'I enjoy the knitting group. I've already made some bootees for my grandson. We talk, mind you, more than we knit, and sort out the world's problems.'

▶

- Model making
- Decorating.

### Group setting

- Painting a mural
- Design a room
- Drama – being in a play
- Line dancing
- Writers' workshop
- Book club
- Synchronised swimming
- Knitting group
- Textiles club
- Ballroom dancing
- Planting a garden.

## Purpose of creative activities

Care workers recognise that creative activities can have a variety of purposes. These include:

- Therapeutic
- Remedial
- Creative
- Intellectual stimulation
- Medical
- Skills for living.

- **Therapeutic** – Healing and restoring to health. For example, painting and writing can be emotionally therapeutic as they express our feelings.
- **Remedial** – Correcting or improving upon an existing skill. For example, a young homeless person will not have had much opportunity to practise cooking. Remedial support will involve providing opportunities to develop this living skill. A young woman who has Down's syndrome may have poor physical co-ordination and remedial support would help to provide opportunities to develop this.
- **Medical** – Someone with a heart condition may have been advised to take some light exercise to increase heart and lung capacity.

## How to select creative activities to suit service users' needs: matching need to activities

The care worker should be aware of the assessment of service users' needs. For example, the autistic child in a special school will have a range of needs involving:

- **Emotional needs** – Difficulty expressing emotions and forming relationships; expresses frustration and rage in ways that are distressing
- **Physical needs** – Inappropriate behaviour towards other children
- **Social needs** – Little need to communicate with others
- **Care needs** – Needs close, personal supervision: no concept of danger
- **Intellectual needs** – Repetitive actions.

The care worker will use this information to choose a creative activity that will target some of these needs. The care worker may decide to develop the service user's social skills by devising creative activities that involve group play.

**Case Study**

Mrs Bolam is an elderly woman in her seventies whose husband has recently died. She suffers from arthritis. Lonely and sad because of her husband's death, she is becoming increasingly isolated. Because of her arthritis she finds it difficult to move around.

*What are Mrs Bolam's physical, intellectual, emotional and social needs?*

*Which creative activities would you choose to meet her needs? Give your reasons.*

Care workers may also need to take into account the service user's interests, hobbies, creative skills and opportunities for creative activities. It would be helpful to think of a variety of activities and then consult, where possible, the service user or if not possible the key worker for that client.

## AO3 Describe the planning process for a creative activity and the importance of the stages within the programme planning

Part of the assessment for this unit is to design and plan a creative activity for use with a service user and to demonstrate an awareness of how this task could be adapted for a different service user.

Before you begin:

- Choose a health, social care or early years setting that provides creative activities for service users and arrange to visit and observe the creative activities on offer.
- Get to know your chosen service user, his/her interests and needs and let them get to know you so that you can build upon a relationship based on respect and trust.

● Prepare witness statements in advance. These must be collected from care staff (giving their professional status) and the service users collected at different stages of the process, signed and dated.

● Keep a diary of your own observations and reflections on the progress of the creative activity.

## Range of activities

Select and agree an appropriate creative activity with your chosen service user. You will need to specify in your process plan whether this creative activity is an individual or a group activity. Give reasons for this choice. The decision to select an individual or group activity will also be based on the assessment you make of your service user's needs. This will be a comprehensive profile of their physical, intellectual, emotional and social needs. You will also need to reference any other relevant information. If for example your service user has had a stroke you will need to research this condition. You will also need to specify the care setting as this will impact upon the way you schedule and deliver the creative activity.

The planning process so far is represented in the flow diagram below.

*Process of planning a creative activity for service users*

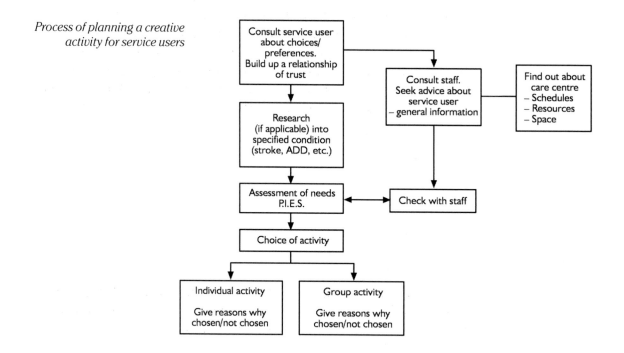

## Aims, objectives and targets

Aims, objectives and targets are important in the planning process as they enable the care worker to think carefully about the value of each part of the creative process to the service user and to assess the overall effectiveness of the plan.

The Aim could be

- To assist the service user in choosing and carrying out a creative activity.

The Objectives could be

- To create a stimulating creative environment
- To encourage and develop the creative abilities of the service user
- To provide an outlet for emotions and feelings in a supportive environment
- To encourage social interaction in a friendly and caring environment.

The Targets would be specific to the physical, intellectual, emotional and social needs of the client. For example:

- To provide opportunities to develop hand/eye co-ordination.

## The importance of identifying the resources required

Once you have decided upon your chosen creative activity you can then proceed to make a list of all the resources you will need. It is important to do this because all the required resources must be available and assembled well in advance to ensure the smooth running of the event. If any problems occur at this stage you can make plans to overcome them and think of alternatives. If after this unforeseen problems occur, consider them positively as learning experiences and write about them in a diary or your evaluation of your own performance.

The resources you need will be:

- Human
- Material
- Time
- Cost.

### Human resources

There may be many people you can access in the course of planning for this activity. As part of your research you may contact a variety of agencies and individuals to help you to understand specific conditions and needs.

- Service user
- Members of the group if a group activity has been selected
- Care centre staff, who will give you clearance to carry out the activity and arrange for a venue to be available
- The caretaker or household manager may need to be consulted. For example, it may be necessary to clear a space of heavy equipment to give you extra room, or simply to make sure of health and safety.

### Material resources

This includes all materials necessary for the creative process. For example, for painting you will need paper, paint, water, jugs and brushes, paper towels, aprons, access to water and soap. It can also include the use of protective clothing such as aprons.

### Time

You will need to know:

- How long the activity will last
- How long it will take to set up
- How long it will take to clear up
- At what time the activity is to take place
- How long it will take you to get to the care counter.

During the activity, keep a record of the time you actually needed and see if it matches the time you planned that it would take to carry out the activity.

### Cost

All care centres work to a strict budget and the cost implications of activities need to be thoroughly explored to see if they are cost-effective. Some care centres may already have the materials you need and allow you to use them. Check different retailers to compare prices and find out suppliers who are the best value for money. Where necessary, improvise. Costumes for acting out a story can be second-hand or from the costume box and this will cost you nothing.

Set yourself a budget, make a note of all costs and see if you can stay within the available budget.

## Importance of protecting service users from harm and maintaining health and safety

Service users in care settings are often vulnerable – physically, emotionally, socially or intellectually. There are laws designed to help protect service users from harm, such as the Children Act 1989, the Care Standards Act 2000 and Health and Safety laws. In addition, all care centres will have in place their own guidelines about how service users are to be protected.

Care workers will already have been screened through the police disclosure process. Staff who are later found to be unsuitable to work with vulnerable adults are referred for possible inclusion on the Protection of Vulnerable Adults register.

You will need to be very careful about the human resources that you use. Seek guidance and clearance from care workers in the care setting.

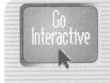

**Find out about the Public Interest Disclosure Act 1998 – visit the Disclosure website:**

- **www.disclosure.gov.uk**

**Find out about the disclosure process, which is necessary to enable someone to work in care settings.**

## Legislation relating to health and safety

The main act relating to health and safety at work is the Health and Safety at Work Act 1974 (HSW Act). This is the umbrella legislation under which all other health and safety laws are made.

These laws recognise the importance of protecting health and safety of staff, service users and others (including visitors) and the management of the safety of equipment, the workplace environment and lifting and handling, among other things. There have been additions to the legislation, such as the Provision and Use of Work Equipment Regulations 1992, but the fundamental issues are set out in the HSW Act.

The Control of Substances Hazardous to Health Regulations 1988 (COSHH) recognises that some chemicals and substances can pose a threat to health and safety.

The Reporting of Injuries, Diseases and Dangerous Occurrences Regulations 1985 (RIDDOR) outlines the procedures for reporting accidents and diseases.

There are some implications for anyone carrying out a creative activity in a care setting. It is advisable to carry out a brief risk assessment to make sure you are aware of any health and safety issues that might be involved in the activity. Here are some brief examples:

### Equipment

- If the equipment is electrical, have the plug and switch been safely checked recently by a qualified safety inspector?
- Is the equipment in good repair and safe to use?
- Can the equipment be safely transported and stored?

### Location

- Is there adequate ventilation?
- Safety – are the windows safe?
- Are Fire Procedures in place?

### Human resources

- Are the people working with you in good health (e.g. do not have flu)?
- Has everybody been police-checked?

### Material resources

Make sure all the materials you are planning to use:

- Do not contain dangerous chemicals (e.g. a child with asthma may be affected)
- Are not infested (e.g. fleas in second-hand costumes).

## Emergencies

Emergencies can occur because of accidents or illness. There will be procedures in place for dealing with accidents and emergencies and care workers will need to know about these. In particular, they will need to know who is the appointed (named) First Aid worker. The method used to deal with any emergency must comply with RIDDOR (1985) and there will be an accident book where all incidents must be recorded.

## Importance of setting criteria for measuring the success of the activity

Criteria are conditions or a set of expectations to be met before a measurement, decision or evaluation be made. The measurement in this case is success and this can be quite difficult to assess. To help with this, it is important to set criteria before carrying out the activity so that you can effectively plan for success and try to build it into the process.

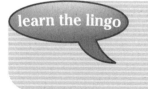

**learn the lingo**

**Criteria** (one is called a **criterion**) are conditions or a set of expectations that must be met before a measurement, decision or evaluation is made.

Here are some criteria for a creative activity that you might find useful:

- The activity is conducted safely
- The service user gets something out of it
- Your own expectations are met
- Resources turn out to be useful and appropriate to the task
- The planning process and organisation is workable
- The service user wants to continue to explore his/her creative talents.

## Values in care

Values in care are well established and include: promoting individual rights and beliefs, maintaining confidentiality, promoting equality and diversity. These are discussed more fully elsewhere in the book.

Table 13.1 lists some examples to help you apply care values when carrying out a creative activity.

*Table 13.1 Care values when carrying out a creative activity*

| Care values | Application |
|---|---|
| Promoting individual rights, beliefs | Choice – service user's wishes: e.g. service user's wishes to be respected e.g. service user chooses the creative activity Belief system: e.g. some religions observe a dress code and service users must be allowed to follow this e.g. a Muslim girl must be able to cover her head |
| Maintaining confidentiality | Do not give other people information about service users |
| Promoting equality and diversity | e.g. a service user who has a disability and is in a wheelchair must still be given a part in a play and access to a full range of creative activities |

## AO4  Plan and carry out a creative activity for an individual

This is a brief outline of planning and carrying out a creative activity.

### Creative activity chosen

- Movement to music (dance).

### Needs of service user

- Service user identified as having attention deficit disorder (ADD)
- Needs identified as intellectual developmental delay for his age (11 years), poor physical co-ordination and muscle control and poor attention span
- Poor self-image.

### Benefits to be gained from creative activity

Physical

- Improve balance, opportunity to develop co-ordination, improve flow of movement (smooth instead of jerky).

## Intellectual

- Listen to and carry out a sequence of movement
- Remember the sequence order
- Improve concentration.

## Emotional

- Raise self-esteem as service user becomes more confident about skills
- Have fun, enjoyment
- Encourage expression of feelings through dance
- Respond emotionally to the music.

## Social

- Not applicable.

## Carry out a creative activity

### Timescales

You need to plan the time in your session carefully. For example, time must be allowed for setting up the activity and also for clearing away.

| Time | Activity |
| --- | --- |
| 12:00 | Collect cassette recorder and tape<br>Open up the room<br>Change into gym clothes |
| 12:15 | Service user arrives |
| 12:20 | Session starts<br>Listen to music chosen, setting the scene |
| 12:25 | Demonstrate to service user a range of movements<br>Reinforce movements by showing a range of flashcards |
| 12:30 | Service user chooses a range of movements |
| 12:35 | Sequence the chosen range of movements |
| 12:40 | Practise movements to music |
| 12:45 | Discuss movements chosen and whether service user feels they work in connection with the music |
| 12:50 | Practise any changes in movements |
| 12:55 | Final run through |
| 13:00 | Close of session |

## Tasks involved within the creative activity

How to do the activity

- Physically demonstrate a range of possible movements to service user
- Show pictures of each movement
- Choose movements, from a range demonstrated, to put together in a dance routine
- Service user to choose and choreograph movement to music
- Service user chooses music.

How the activity will be carried out

- Individual activity
- Service user working with student.

## Plan and organise resources for the activity

Human resources

- Service user
- Student (Health and Social Care: Intermediate)
- Teacher of Special Needs (when necessary).

Material resources

- Gym clothes/track suit or own clothes
- Music tapes
- Cassette recorder.

Time

- Dinnertime 12:20–13:00.

Cost

- Nil (own tape, small recorder).

## Put in timescales

Aim

- To enable the service user to move creatively to music of his choice.

Objectives

- To provide opportunities for creative self-expression
- To provide a sense of achievement and raise self-esteem
- To help service user build productive relationships with others.

CREATIVE ACTIVITIES WITH INDIVIDUALS IN CARE SETTINGS

Targets

- To increase attention span
- To help intellectual development – memorising sequences
- To help promote flowing physical movements.

### Set pre-set criteria for measuring the success of the activity

These could include:

- Carry out the creative activity safely
- Service user enjoys the activity
- Good relationships built up with service user
- Develop my own communication skills
- Complete the task and achieve some or all of the objectives
- Fulfil organiser's expectations – happy at final outcome.

### Health and safety requirements

- Awareness of fire drill procedures in care setting – for service users and visitors
- Knowledge of location of nearest exit point in case of fire
- Check the floor in the school gym is not dirty or slippery and has no debris on it
- Check temperature of room
- Make sure all electrical equipment has been safety checked.

### Applying the value base in care

You need to describe details of how the value base in care was applied when carrying out the activity. Feedback from the service user will help you to understand your good care. For example:

- Communication – Could you hear my voice?
- Dignity/choice –Were you comfortable doing the movements? Did the service user choose the music?

Witness statements, questionnaires and oral feedback are all important parts of the process both before, during and after carrying out the activity and will help you to assess your application of care values.

## AO5  Evaluate the creative activity

**learn the lingo**

**Evaluate** means to examine or judge something carefully, to work out its value or worth.

426  OCR Level 2 National Certificate in Health and Social Care

The evaluation process can be broken down into four main areas:

- **Reflection** – This means looking carefully back over your work and considering all aspects of your own performance.

- **Analysing** – This means examining in detail, breaking down into parts and judging your own performance. Analysis should involve a growing awareness of your skills and qualities and your strengths and weaknesses.

- **Making informed decisions** – This means making a judgement based on knowledge and information. For example, your service user may not want to join in the planned creative activity. Your knowledge of care values means that you understand that your service user has the right to choose to join in or not, as the case may be.

- **Planning for improvement** – This involves drawing up a plan, or a schedule, where you list all the areas that you need to improve upon. Against each one, explain what action you need to take to improve. You may wish to add a further column that you can tick when you have addressed the issues.

Evaluating the creative activity with service users in care settings will therefore involve measuring, judging and assessing the value of the creative activity to the service user.

It will be helpful to apply the following criteria when looking closely at and assessing the success of the activity:

- Own performance
- Benefits to the service user
- Relationship with service users
- Applying the principles of good practice
- Achievement of aims, objectives, targets, costs
- Applying the values of care.

Evaluation is an ongoing process and an important part of the care worker's role in providing quality care for the service user. It also helps the care worker to recognise and build upon good practice. Evaluation can be self-evaluation but assessments, witness statements and feedback from others, including the service user, can also provide valuable information advice, and can thus enhance the evaluation process.

## Own performance

Evaluating your own performance involves looking carefully at and reviewing how you approached the task and how you demonstrated your ability to plan, prepare and participate in a creative activity for a service user. You will need to examine the quality and relevance of the research you made into the needs of the service user, and judge how well you matched the creative activity to the needs you identified.

You will need to identify your own skills and qualities, including practical skills such as organisation and time planning, as well as personal qualities such as patience and sensitivity. You will have found out much about yourself during this activity, and may also be able to identify your own strengths and weaknesses together with areas of professional expertise that you can share with others and areas that you understand you need to develop further.

## Benefits to the service user

The benefits to the service user may be physical, intellectual, emotional and/or social. You will need to refer back to the needs (P.I.E.S.) of the service user and decide whether these needs have been met. For example, an older service user in a care setting who has arthritis may have found the gentle movement to music programme helpful in easing painful joints and maintaining mobility. This is a physical benefit. Equally, an autistic child may have allowed you to work alongside him/her while painting, and this may be considered a social and emotional benefit.

## Relationship with service users

Caring for others involved building relationships that are rewarding both for the carer and the service user. The service user has a valuable part to play in the evaluation. Consult the service user about his/her thoughts and feelings throughout the creative programme. You may have kept a log or diary, and reflecting on this will help you assess how your relationship with the service user has developed. You may devise a simple questionnaire that service users can respond to and this can also give you an indication of how he/she felt the relationship developed. You could also ask a careworker to observe you interacting with the service user, and then talk through their observations with you.

## Applying the principles of good practice

The principles of good care are as follows:

- Maintaining confidentiality
- Being sensitive to the needs of individuals
- Communicating effectively
- Promoting and supporting individuals' rights to dignity, independence and choice.

Line managers, supervisors and ward sisters are among a few of those who could contribute to the assessment of your professional conduct. You could devise a tick-list or a questionnaire where your communication skills, interpersonal skills and your sensitivity to the service users could be assessed.

## Achievement of aims, objectives, targets, costs

Look carefully at the aims, objectives, targets and costs that you outlined at the beginning of the project. Describe carefully whether they were achieved or not. Where you did not fully achieve an aim, objective or target, try to explain why.

## Applying the values of care

Values of care underpin all aspects of care work. The care values common to the full range of service users are:

- Promoting individual rights and beliefs
- Maintaining confidentiality
- Promoting equality and diversity.

Students who have worked with children will need to extend this list to include early years care values. These include the above values, in addition to the following:

- The welfare of the child
- Maintaining a healthy and safe environment
- Working with others
- Helping the child to meet their full potential.

In your evaluation you will need to describe fully how you upheld each care value. Try to give one example of good practice for each. Also comment on the values of care that you were unable to meet fully.

## AO6 Describe how the activity could be adapted for a service user with different needs

It is useful in care practice to be able to modify and adapt plans of work to suit the needs of alternative service users.

Below are some examples of how the plan could be adopted to meet the needs of an elderly lady with impaired physical ability in a care home.

### Adaptations

#### Needs of service user

Physical needs

- Poor muscle tone
- Poor heart and lung capacity
- Stiff joints
- Easily tired.

Emotional needs

- Is depressed because she is not as mobile as she used to be

Intellectual needs

No need to adapt.

Social needs

Not applicable.

## The activity: adaptations

The care worker will have to choose a different set of movements that are easier to do and less physically demanding. Some of these movements – or all – may take place while the service user is sitting. The movements will need to be based around physical movements the service user is capable of. A care worker will need to be present or nearby in case of emergencies. The service user will need to wear loose clothing to allow for easier movement.

Some of the objectives and targets will need to be adapted.

Objectives could include:

- To provide opportunities for social interaction with others
- To bring a sense of enjoyment and fulfilment
- To give an outlet for emotional feelings and so help with the service user's sense of depression
- To give a feeling of physical well-being and a positive 'can-do' attitude

Targets could include:

- To help develop muscle tone
- To build up strength so that the service user does not tire so easily.

### Resources

- Different music will need to be selected for an elderly person.

### Costs

- Will remain the same.

### Time

- This will be different, as dinner time is not an appropriate time to carry out a creative activity with an elderly person. Ask the service user and seek advice from care staff about the most appropriate time in the care home's schedule.
- Several short sessions, each for example of 20 minutes, may be another adaptation that can be made. The service user is likely to tire easily, and this needs to be taken into account.

**further information**

Evans K and Dubowski J (2001) *Art Therapy with Children on the Autistic Spectrum.* Jessica Kingsley, London

www.asbah.org – Association for Spina Bifida

www.cftrust.org.uk – Cystic Fibrosis Trust

www.dfsg.org.uk – Duchenne Family Support

www.dsa-uk.com – Down's Syndrome Association

www.dyspraxiafoundation.org.uk – British Dyspraxia Foundation

www.epilepsy.org.uk – Epilepsy Action

www.epilepsynse.org.uk – National Society for Epilepsy

www.fragilex.org.uk – Fragile X Society

www.hacsg.org.uk – Hyperactive Children

www.hse.gov.uk/coshh – Health and Safety Executive

www.look-uk.org – National Federation for the Visually Impaired

www.nas.org.uk – National Autistic Society

www.ndcs.org.uk – National Deaf Children's Society

www.scope.org.uk – SCOPE

## Summary

- Creative activities (e.g. dancing, writing, knitting) provide benefits to service users in a number of physical, intellectual, environmental and social ways.

- Creative activities and their purposes could vary from swimming, which may have the medical purpose of helping to ease arthritic pain, to creative writing, which may have the therapeutic purpose of allowing a service user to express their feelings.

- When planning a creative activity for a particular service user it is important to get to know them and their needs and involve them in the planning if possible. Availability of resources needed – people, materials, time and cost – must be considered.

- When carrying out a creative activity, it is a good idea to keep a record of the outcomes, planned benefits and timescales allowed to evaluate the activity's success.

- An activity could be adapted for another service user, for example a physical activity could be made up of less demanding movements and/ or the activity could be moved to a group setting where the focus is on social interaction for the service user.

# Glossary

**ABC procedures**: A sequential emergency first aid process – Airway, Breathing, Circulation

**Accurate records**: Factual records kept by the setting following an accident or concern

**Active listening**: Ensuring that you are focusing on what you are listening to

**Acute disability**: A condition that occurs suddenly, which may be severe and may last for a relatively short time. Examples are a broken leg or arm

**Advocacy**: Representing another individual or speaking on their behalf

**Aggressive**: Taking a forceful approach

**Assertive**: Able to put your ideas or viewpoint across without aggression

**Balanced diet**: A diet that provides a person with enough of the various types of nutrient to meet their needs. It does not have excesses (too much) or deficiencies (too little) of anything

**Barriers to communication**: Any obstruction to understanding between individuals

**Basic physical needs**: Needs humans have that must be met in order for them to stay alive. These include the need for shelter and the needs to satisfy hunger, thirst and sexual desire. They include also the need to maintain temperature, the need for oxygen, sleep and sensory pleasure

**Body language**: The non-verbal signals given out by our bodies

**Braille**: Words written as a series of raised dots, read by some people with visual impairment

**Care of the environment**: Considering the safety needs of the early years setting

**Care values**: The principles, standards or qualities considered worthwhile and desirable by the care profession. It is important that people working in the health and care professions hold these values and apply them in their work. These professionals are described as working from the care values

**Chiropodist**: A trained professional who looks after people's feet

**Chronic disability**: A condition that develops slowly over a long period or lasts a long time, often a condition that is incurable, such as chronic arthritis

**Closed questions**: Questions that place a limit on the possible answers

**Communication**: Passing and receiving information from one person to another and back

**Compulsory referral**: The admission to care or hospital of someone against their will. People who are considered a danger to themselves or who are mentally ill may be compulsorily referred to hospital for care

**Confidentiality**: Keeping information to yourself; not passing on information inappropriately

**Congenital disability**: A condition that exists at birth but is not necessarily inherited

**Continuity of care**: Routine and familiarity, which helps children feel secure

**COSHH**: Control of Substances Hazardous to Health

**Cross-infection**: The passing of infection from one person to another

**Development**: The changes that take place as an individual grows

**Developmental delay**: The term often used when a child's development is not following the pattern of averages

**Direct discrimination**: Treating people less favourably than others because of their gender, race, disability, etc.

**Disclosure**: Telling someone about the abuse suffered, either currently or in the past

**Discrimination**: What a person does – how they treat another person or group unfairly, based on their prejudice

**Droplet infection**: A common cause of cross-infection

**Emotional needs**: Need for love, to be wanted, to be respected

**Empowerment**: Enabling people to make decisions for themselves

**Equality**: The state of being equal, of having an equal opportunity

**Equity**: Fairness combined with equal opportunity

**Evaluation**: Reflecting on and giving consideration to a past event, action or project

**First aid**: The emergency actions taken following an accident or sudden illness

**Health promotion**: Advising others about health and well-being. Health promotion materials such as videos and pamphlets may help to get the message across

**Identifying needs**: Being able to recognise a need using professional judgement, knowledge and understanding

**Indirect discrimination**: Where conditions are set that exclude certain groups – for example a requirement that all police wear uniform hats will exclude Sikhs who wear turbans

**Lifestyle factors**: The impact of lifestyle choices such as smoking, diet, age, exercise and sleep that have an impact on health

**Menopause**: Stage of a woman's life involving a series of hormone changes. This eventually means the end of the woman's ability to have children

**National Curriculum**: The curriculum followed by children in all state schools

**Natural immunity**: A degree of immunity present in the body without the use of vaccination

**Nutritionally deficient**: Lacking the correct levels of vitamins and minerals for a healthy body

**Obese**: Very overweight, to the extent of risking health

**Observation skills**: The ability to carry out appropriate methods of observation, knowing when to use them and how

**Open questions**: Questions that encourage a detailed answer

**Paraphrasing**: Restating what you have heard someone else say; used to clarify understanding

**Personal space**: The space that a person needs for themselves, where only those they know well can enter. You shake hands with people you have just met, but you may let others into your personal space and hug them

**Personality**: Aspects of a person's character that remain relatively permanent

**Physical environment**: The surroundings ,building, room layout, lighting, ventilation

**Physical needs**: Physical needs include food, sleep, warmth, sex and shelter

**Poor personal hygiene**: Not washing the hands, body, hair and teeth properly. This causes the spread of more disease than anything else in the care sector

**Potential hazard**: Any situation which has the potential to cause harm

**Primary Care Team**: The first call when a person needs a health or care service. The team includes general practitioners (GPs), nurses, social workers and support workers, such as home carers

**Primary Health Care Trusts**: Trusts that plan and deliver local health care services such as general practitioner services, hospitals and community nursing services

**Professional referral**: When a person is put in touch with a service by a doctor, social worker, nurse, teacher or when other professionals assist the person to request care

**Protein**: A nutrient found in food. It is used to build and repair cells and tissues

**Psychosocial**: Describing problems or issues that affect a person's mental or psychological state as well as affecting their relationships and social contacts

**Puberty**: Age of 'adulthood', when physical changes occur in the body because of the increased production of the sex hormones oestrogen in girls and testosterone in boys

**Pulse rate**: A measure of the heart rate. The average pulse rate is about 70 beats per minute

**Recovery position**: The position individuals are placed in following an accident or sudden illness, after their situation has been stabilised, while they await further medical treatment

**Referral procedures**: The process of reporting concerns about a service user's safety

**Reflective listening**: Where the listener echoes the last words spoken by the speaker

**Respiratory**: Concerned with breathing

**Risks to health**: Anything that might have a negative effect upon a person's health. These things can be physical, social, emotional or intellectual and include poor diet, changing jobs, loss or bereavement or stress

**Sedentary**: Literally, sitting around. Used to describe someone who does not take much exercise or a job that involves sitting down most of the day

**Self-awareness**: Understanding of how you are perceived by others and the impact you have on them

**Self-concept**: Describes the way we see and think about ourselves. This includes not only our physical appearance but also our understanding of what kind of person we are

**Self-esteem**: Describes how we value ourselves. Self-esteem is a value judgement we hold about ourselves, which evaluates ourselves in relation to our own and others' expectations

**Self-referral**: The term used when people seek help themselves. This may involve support from family members

**Statutory service**: Service set up by the government under legislation (law). Examples are the National Health Service and Social Services Departments

**Strategic Health Authorities**: New health authorities that replaced the old district health authorities. Strategic Health Authorities have a number of key jobs:

Find out the health needs of the local population

Develop a strategy for meeting those needs

Decide what services are necessary to meet local needs

Allocate resources (money) to Primary Care Trusts

Make sure that Primary Care Trusts work properly

**Tertiary health care**: Ongoing care of chronic conditions, often by specialist community-based health professionals

# Index

Page references in *italics* indicate tables or diagrams. Those in **bold** indicate where terms have been defined.

Hygiene
  babies 227–32
  care settings 105–32
  children 136, 261–2, *262*
  food 116–17
  oral 112
Hyperthermia 144–5, 182
Hypothermia 182

Imaginative play 267
Indirect discrimination 14, 23, **434**
Individual care plans 27–8
Individual rights 7–8, 10, 11–12, 63, 75–6
Infection
  prevention 110–6
  risk 106–9
  spread of 105–9, *114*
  vaccination 108
Information
  exchange of 42
Insecurity 218
Intellectual activities
  and older people 193–4
Intellectual development
  of infant 209–15, *210–2*
Intellectual needs 137, *245*
  challenge 246
  stimulation 245
  and older people 170–4, 285–6
Interpersonal
  communication 78
  interaction 51–3
  skills 77, **247**
Interviews 31–7
Involuntary movements **206**
Irritable bowel syndrome 392–3

Language 42
Layette **230**, *231*
Learning difficulties 409
Legislation 19, 21–7
  health and safety 259–61, 350–2, 421–2
Life expectancy **162**, *163*
Lifestyle **435**
  and health 165–6
  and pregnancy 204
Lifting equipment *91*
Listening 53–4, 60–2,78
Long Term Care Charter 3
Looking-on play 265
Lower reference nutrient intake (LRNI)
  379
Lung volume 154

Makaton 59–60, *60*
Manipulative play 267
Manual Handling Operations Regulations
  92, 351
Maslow's theory of human needs 169–70,
  *169*, 282–3, *283*
Meals-on-wheels 180, 279

Medicines 143
  disposal 115
  safety 137
  storage 130–1
Mental health 410–11
  older people 286
Mental Health Act Commission 23
Microbes 105–6
  multiplication of *106*
Midwife 223
MIND 6
Mineral deficiencies 390–1
Mission statements 26–7
Mobility
  aids *89*, 89–93
  benefits of 88–9
Mouth-to-mouth resuscitation 359–60
MRSA (Methicillin–Resistant
  Staphylococcus Aureus) 109
Muscular dystrophy 135

National Association of Citizens' Advice
  Bureaux 6
National Disability Council 5
National Health Service and Community
  Care Act 1990 24
Natural immunity **226**, **435**
Nature/nurture 244
Newborn *225*
  bathing 229–30
  care needs 223
  clothes 230–2
  equipment for 232–5, *232*, 206–8
  formalities 224–5
  nappy changing 227–8
  nappy rash 228–9
  professionals 223–4
  reflex actions *206*
  tests on 225
Non-starch polysaccharide (NSP) 388
Non-verbal communication 46, 56–60
  and babies *212*
Nursery nurse 248
Nursery schools 238
Nursery teacher 249–50
Nursery
  designing 233–5, *234*
  equipment *232*, 232–3
  safety *253*
Nutrient groups *386*
Nutrient Triangle *199*
Nutritional deficiencies 389–92, **435**
Nutritional requirements 380–4
  adults *381*, 400–1
  babies 384
  children 382–3, 400, 401
  culture 384–5
  older people *381*, 400, 402
  pregnant women 383
  teenagers *382*
  vegetarians 384, 400, 402

440 *OCR Level 2 National Certificate in Health and Social Care*

Observation 31, **435**
Occupational therapists 281
Older people
  communicating with 296–9
  cultures 167
  eating patterns 399
  family 166
  health provision 280–2
  helping 305–7
  hospitalisation 180–1
  illnesses 182
  loneliness 166
  media 167
  needs of 168–74
  nutritional requirements 380–1, *381*
  perceptions of 166
  personal care 278, 286–7
  recreation 307–12
  service provision 274–9, *275*
  support workers 174–81, *177*
Open questions 52–3, 297, **435**
Oral hygiene 112
Osteoporosis 184–5

Paediatricians 142
Parallel play 265
Paraphrasing 53–4, 298, **435**
Parent-held records 226
Parents
  influence of 244
  responsibilities 198–205, *199*
Peak flow 190–1, *190*, **191**
Personal hygiene 82–4
  aids for 87–8, *88*
Personal rights 7–8
Personal space **57, 435**
Physical activities 154–5
  and older people 193
Physical development 205–9, **206**
  aged 1–3, 208–9, *208*
  of infant *207*
Physical disabilities 325–6, 409
Physical environment 46, **435**
Physical needs 136, **435**
  of children *243*
  and older people 169, 170, 282–3, 284–5
Physical play 267
Physical rights 8
Physiotherapist 175, 280
PIES *266*
PKU test 225
Play 137–8, *222*
  and development 221
  role of 264
  stages of 265–6
  types of 266–8
Playgroups 239
  leader 248–9
Policies **20**
Positive positioning 57–8
Postnatal care 140, 223

Preconceptual care 198–9
Pregnancy
  clothing 202–3
  diet 96–7, *199*, 199–200
  emotions 203
  exercise 201–2, *201*
  father's role 204–5
  physical changes 203–4, *204*
Prescriptive **55**
Procedures **20**
  explaining 42
Prompting 53
Prone position 358
Protective clothing 111
Protein 385–6, **436**
Public authorities 25
Pulse **436**
  errors 153
  measuring 148–9, *148*, 190

Qualities **247**, *247*
Questioning 51, 297
Questionnaires 31–7

Race Relations Acts 22–3
Racial discrimination 14
Recovery position 357, *358*, **436**
Reference nutrient intake (RNI) 378, 395, *396*
Referral **329, 436**
Reflective listening 54, **436**
Reflex actions *206*
Relationships
  promoting 43, 45–6
  secure 244
Report
  writing 37
Residential provision 276–7
Respiratory arrest 357
Respiratory rate 154
Respiratory system conditions 186
Rheumatism 184
RIDDOR (Reporting of Injuries, Diseases and Danger Occurances Regulations) 1995 112–13, 263–4
Rights 1–3
  Financial 8
  Individual 7–8, 10, 11–12
  Personal 7–8
  Physical 8
  Removal of 20–1
Risk **119**
  assessment 255–7, **257**, 294–5, **294**, 345–53
  reducing 122–3

Safety audit 347, 349–50
Safety needs 136
  and older people 169, 171–2, 283
Safety surveys 122